Design Thinking in Healthcare

Anni Pakarinen • Thomas Lemström
Eeva Rainio • Eriikka Siirala
Editors

Design Thinking in Healthcare

From Problem to Innovative Solutions

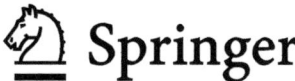 Springer

Editors
Anni Pakarinen (iD)
Faculty of Medicine
Department of Nursing Science
University of Turku
Turku, Finland

Eeva Rainio (iD)
Faculty of Medicine
University of Turku
Turku, Finland

Thomas Lemström
SPARK Finland
Turku, Finland

Eriikka Siirala (iD)
Faculty of Medicine
University of Turku
Turku, Finland

ISBN 978-3-031-24509-1   ISBN 978-3-031-24510-7   (eBook)
https://doi.org/10.1007/978-3-031-24510-7

This Springer imprint is published by the registered company Springer Nature Switzerland AG
The registered company address is: Gewerbestrasse 11, 6330 Cham, Switzerland

Preface

Healthcare managers of the past viewed patients' needs merely as targets for population-level health outcomes to be validated in the final phases of developing interventions and services. Today, we know better. Patients' needs and experiences should be viewed as sources of innovation at the front-end of the development process. It provides the basis for applying design thinking to develop better healthcare services and health tech applications.

Today, the success of any healthcare service depends on complex interactions between various stakeholders, and new solutions can only be delivered effectively through co-creative and collaborative efforts. Coordinating such efforts relies on strong concepts that can only result from properly run design processes that this book describes in light of case studies around the world.

Design thinking is receiving increasing attention in the field, as forward-thinking organizations delve into the practice. It can change the way medical solutions are created and how clinical services are delivered. By driving innovation by means of empathy and practicality, design thinking provides tools for those seeking to drive radical renewal in the field.

Design thinking is crucial generalist skill, and this book presents design thinking for nurses and other healthcare professionals, researchers, students, and educators to support their development as creative and transformative leaders in their fields.

Turku, Finland	Anni Pakarinen
Turku, Finland	Thomas Lemström
Turku, Finland	Eeva Rainio
Turku, Finland	Eriikka Siirala

Contents

1   Why Design Thinking Matters in Healthcare   1
    Anni Pakarinen

2   Ethical Aspects and Innovations in Healthcare   9
    Helena Siipi and Mari Kangasniemi

3   Design Thinking Toolkit for Healthcare Innovation 25
    Beate Rygg Johnsen

4   Design Thinking in Healthcare Education 37
    Isabella Hajduk, Annika Nordberg, and Eeva Rainio

5   Design Thinking Driven Solutions for Health 63
    Janne Pühvel, Janne Kommusaar, and Annika Nordberg

6   Using Design Thinking in Nursing Management
    and Leadership 79
    Eriikka Siirala, Outi Tuominen, and Sanna Salanterä

7   Co-creation and Change in Healthcare. 91
    Laura Niemi

8   New Business Creation in Health Technology 101
    Kaapo Seppälä

9   What is the Importance of Design Thinking
    for Future Healthcare?. 113
    Thomas Lemström

Editors and Contributors

About the Editors

Anni Pakarinen is a registered nurse and has a PhD in Health Sciences. Pakarinen works as a senior researcher and research manager in the Department of Nursing Science, University of Turku, Finland. Her research focuses on health promotion and digital interventions, particularly on serious games and gamified applications. She leads several digital health projects and is experienced in developing, evaluating, and implementing interventions for health. During recent years, she has been involved in planning and organizing several international and multiprofessional design thinking courses at the University of Turku.

Thomas Lemström works as a business design advisor for teams creating new products, services, and content that drive innovative change in healthcare. His experiences in the field include founding a biotech company, running an accelerator program for innovative health and wellness solutions, consulting in healthcare management, and serving as a business design advisor for researchers and developers of medical technologies.

Eeva Rainio has a PhD in Molecular Biology, and she has been working in university administration since 2010, first in MSc and doctoral program coordination, and then with strategic development, innovations, and business collaboration. She has also played a significant role in introducing design thinking to the Faculty of Medicine at the University of Turku, after her visit to Stanford d.school in 2019.

Eriikka Siirala is a registered nurse and has a PhD in Health Sciences. Her research focuses on nurse managers decision-making and information needs in perioperative settings. At the moment, Siirala works as a chief innovation specialist in the wellbeing services county of Southwest Finland. In addition, she also works part-time in the Faculty of Medicine at the university of Turku. Siirala got inspired to use design thinking after a visit to Stanford d.school, and she has been involved in design thinking courses at the university and also in the hospital.

About the Contributors

Isabella Hajduk is a microbiologist, who undertook her PhD at the University of Technology Sydney (UTS) in Australia. She teaches Biomedical Innovation and Entrepreneurship course and Innovation, Entrepreneurship and Commercialization (IEC) as a Master's subject at UTS. In Isabella's courses, biomedical sciences are successfully combined with design thinking approach.

Mari Kangasniemi is working as a professor and the Vice Head of the Department of Nursing Science in the University of Turku, Finland and as a Visiting Professor at the University of Tartu, Estonia. She has worked at the university as a full-time researcher and teacher since 2002. Her main research interest has been focused on nursing and healthcare ethics, and she is also investigating the change of social and healthcare work and environmental responsibility in patient care. Kangasniemi acts as a research group leader, is a member of national and international multidisciplinary research groups, is supervisor and teacher for academic degrees, and is the lecturer and expert in various scientific and societal groups and tasks.

Janne Kommusaar has an MSc in Health Sciences (Nursing Science). Kommusaar works as a responsible teacher of nursing pedagogy courses for Nursing Science master's students at the University of Tartu. Before her academic career, she worked as a school nurse and a nurse in the surgery department. Kommusaar has always been interested in new technologies and how to utilize these in education and healthcare. She was involved in an international project where design thinking online and intensive course were created and implemented for multidisciplinary students to solve diverse healthcare problems and create innovative and new solutions.

Laura Niemi has a PhD in Entrepreneurship. Her research focuses on the co-creation of new value and touches upon the intersection of strategic management, entrepreneurship, and marketing domains. Now Niemi is working as a Development Specialist at Research Development and Administration unit of the University of Turku. In her current work, Niemi is committed to shaping the ways the research is carried out and communicated in the future, and she is passionate about facilitation, visualization, and bringing strategic thinking closer to the academic leaders and researchers.

Annika Nordberg is a public health nurse and holds a master's degree of Health Sciences from the University of Turku. Annika's passion has always been in the improvement of patients and end users' experience. During her studies, she became acquainted with Stanford Design Thinking process and how to utilize it in the field of healthcare, including health education. She took part in an international intensive training program in the area of Biomedical Innovation and Entrepreneurship (BIE2020) organized by SPARK. After completing the course, she got the opportunity to work for SPARK Finland. She has also coached and organized different customer experience workshops for healthcare professionals.

Janne Pühvel is a university teacher in the Department of Nursing Science, University of Tartu. In 2020–21, she was involved in developing and conducting an international online course about applying design thinking in health technology education. She has previously worked as a nurse in the department of emergency orthopedics and is currently participating in a project aiming to improve the quality and patient safety in surgical care.

Beate Rygg Johnsen is a biochemist from the University of Oslo (UiO) and has built her carrier in a global industry setting. She has worked in biotech, pharma, and the start-up scene with innovation, business strategy, and commercialization. She has broad experience with innovation processes such as IDEO and Design Thinking. In her current positions as senior innovation adviser at UiO, she works to bring some of this knowledge into academia to foster innovation and creative thinking.

Sanna Salanterä is a Vice Dean in the Faculty of Medicine and Professor in Clinical Nursing science in the University of Turku, Finland. Currently, Salanterä's main research intersects are health technology and clinical nursing. Her research team "Connected Health" develops and studies gamification of health, IoT for nursing and health, symptom care, information technology to support clinical decision-making, and text mining of clinical narratives.

Kaapo Seppälä is teaching Software Project Management and Mixed Reality Technologies in the Department of Computing in the University of Turku, Finland. He also works as Sales Lead in a University Spin-off in the company CTRL Reality which is specialized in Mixed Reality B2B products and services. Seppälä has experience in commercialization and selling software products in complex regulatory environments.

Helena Siipi is a Doctor of Social Sciences and Docent of Philosophical Ethics. Siipi works as a University Lecturer in the Department of Philosophy, Contemporary History, and Political Science at the University of Turku, Finland. She obtained her PhD in Philosophy in 2005. She conducts research in applied ethics and environmental philosophy on a wide range of topics including the philosophy of food, the ethics of new biotechnologies and ethical issues related to biodiversity. She has wide teaching experience and her articles have been used as teaching materials at institutions such as Michigan State University and SLU Uppsala. At the University of Turku, Siipi has made a particular contribution as a teacher of research ethics for undergraduate and postgraduate students.

Outi Tuominen, RN, PhD is Nurse Director from the Department of Pediatrics and Adolescent Medicine, Turku University Hospital, Finland. She has over 10 years of management experience. Her Post-Doctoral research interest includes Nursing Leadership, Nursing Management, Patient Safety, and Quality Improvement.

Why Design Thinking Matters in Healthcare

Anni Pakarinen

1.1   Introduction

Design thinking can be viewed as a systematic, iterative, and exploratory innovation process to solve complex problems [1]. It offers an accessible problem-solving and innovation framework and methods to apply when developing new products and services. It may also refer to a way of thinking and approaching issues, in other words considered as a philosophy per se [2, 3]. The success behind many companies is that they have woken up to the requirement of user orientation as they design and develop new products, and in their processes, they utilized design thinking methods and tools to gain with desired, compelling, feasible, and viable end-products [3–5].

Individualistic society has set a basis for the demands of citizens, and this affects not only the need for user-friendly products but also the services that should be tailored according to the needs and preferences of individuals. This development also facilitates the sustainability goals, when instead of producing solutions for society without well-thought reasons and deeper understanding of the users and their needs, we are designing and developing solutions that have real demand and need. This progress may lead to more effective, impactful, and sustainable solutions and produce real value for the whole society [4].

This change has been seen also in the field of healthcare, and the end-users of healthcare products and services—in other words clients, patients, and healthcare professionals—are nowadays in the key role in the whole process of the development. Development cannot happen in isolation. Thus, instead of seeing end-users just as a receiver or producer of care and treatment, we see them as active partners, valuable informants, and sources of innovation to bring value to the whole healthcare [4, 6].

A. Pakarinen (✉)
Faculty of Medicine, Department of Nursing Science, University of Turku, Turku, Finland
e-mail: anni.pakarinen@utu.fi

© The Author(s), under exclusive license to Springer Nature   1
Switzerland AG 2023
A. Pakarinen et al. (eds.), *Design Thinking in Healthcare*,
https://doi.org/10.1007/978-3-031-24510-7_1

The demand for patient, client, and user-centered approach in healthcare provides the basis for applying design thinking to develop better healthcare services and health technology solutions, and provide better experiences to the clients and patients [7, 8]. Thus, design thinking has received increasing attention also in healthcare. One of the main reasons for this is the fact that design thinking emphasizes deep empathy for end-user's perceptions, needs, and challenges [9].

In design thinking process, designers and developers begin with research and empathic engagement with the stakeholders, who are most affected by and knowledgeable about a product and service under development. After empathizing, designers and developers dive deeper to the theme and define the problem for which they then start generating ideas to solve. Last few phases consist of the selection of most feasible idea to produce prototypes and test them among intended end-users [4, 10].

1.2   What Is Design Thinking?

The origins of design thinking ideology lead to a book called *Sciences of the Artificial*, written in 1969 by a political scientist and a receiver of the Nobel Memorial Prize in Economic Sciences, Herbert A. Simon. The design thinking term itself is traced to a book called *Design as a Discipline*, written in 1979 by a mechanical engineer and professor of Design Research, Bruce Archer [11].

Design thinking offers a framework for complex problem solving applied widely by various disciplines. It is traditionally associated with the business, innovation, and customer-oriented development of products and services, where the goal is to gain success, sustainability, and customer benefit. Design thinking has received increased attention in industry, engineering, and architecture, as well as in educational contexts (see Chap. 4). Design thinking can change how people solve problems, but also how they learn, thus offering a favorable soil for success [4, 9, 12].

Design thinking is a term we use, when we are adapting the principles, tools, and methods familiar from design by traditional designers, but use it somewhere else than merely for traditional purposes. Design thinking can be viewed as a systematic, iterative, and exploratory innovation process that puts emphasis into deep empathy for end-user perceptions, needs, and challenges. It also offers methods, aspirations, and a way to see and approach issues form different perspective. In a broader sense, design thinking may be seen as a philosophy. It can be seen as a targeted way to produce the best possible experience for the end-user [11–14].

Design thinking is not only about the design or development of products or services. It can be also seen as team-based process, which allows us to see the whole process of design and development to be as meaningful as the end-product that is designed. The development process is itself a learning experience for the designers, the team who works together for the common goal. Design thinking is therefore often associated with the concept of co-design, which will be discussed further in Chap. 7. The way the team works together—able to combine approaches, perceptions, and views—is relevant. How they find a balance between disagreements, similarities, and different ways of thinking is interesting and the end result is often a reflection of the designers and the balance they have found [12, 15].

1.3   Toward the Solution Following Design Thinking Process

As described above, design thinking offers us with a process to follow when designing and developing user-centered products and services. Depending on the source of design thinking literature, different terminology and definitions exist, and different types of phases of the process may be detected. For example, a recent review found altogether 35 different process models in design thinking. However, the source of the design thinking approach used, the principles, and main idea of end-user engagement are the same [12]. In this chapter we take an approach and model derived from Stanford d.school and adapt their terminology and definitions to describe the design thinking approach [16].

In design thinking process, designers begin with empathic engagement with the stakeholders who are affected by the problem and who have the most experience and knowledge on it. In this first phase, we need deep empathy for end-user perceptions, needs, and challenges to fully understand a problem to come up with more comprehensive, feasible, and viable solutions. After this empathic phase, designers begin a phase that goes beyond the surface to come up with the root cause of the problem. This is when they have a solid basis to create solutions, prototype them, and test them among the users [11, 17, 18].

The first phase of the design thinking process is empathizing, understanding the customer's real needs. Aim of this phase is to get personal grasps of the needs of the users (of the service, device, etc.) and to really understand their experiences, motivations, challenges, and problems. This is done best, when we forget our assumptions and begin to obtain insights into the world of the users. To truly solve a problem, we must have an empathetic view of the people who experience that problem. Users have a wealth of first-hand knowledge of what works and what doesn't, which we should use as an advantage. During this phase the empathetic view is taken by observing and consulting with users. For example, we can do a literature review on the given topic, explore statistics on the problem and its occurrence, extent and frequency among population to find out the people that a problem mainly has an effect on. This phase may not be limited to exploring previous studies, but also exploring how, when, and why it affects the people. Thus, empirical studies are also suggested, such as survey studies and interviews among the stakeholders [4, 13, 19].

The second phase of the design thinking process is defining, stating users' perceptions, needs, and problems. Aim of this phase is to interpret and analyze observations (empathizing) and synthesize them to define the core problem. These definitions are called problem statements. You produce insights that form solid foundations for finding solutions. The idea is to dig deeper the problem and see the root causes for the problem. During the defining phase, we focus on the problem to find new ways of doing things. We may adopt different methods to define the problem (see more about design thinking methods from Chap. 3) [4, 13, 17].

The third phase of the design thinking process is ideating. Aim of this phase is to start generating ideas to identify new solutions to the problem you have detected. Idea is to look for alternative ways of viewing and solving the problem. During ideation, it is possible to see beyond the usual methods of solving problems in order to find better, more suitable, and satisfying solutions to problems [4, 11]. To have number of ideas it's crucial to have a team who holds experience and expertise from different fields, the more heterogeneous the team is, the more fruitful and various solutions are created. The team may include the content expertise, but also engineers, IT-experts, marketing, and commercial experts [20].

The fourth phase of the design thinking process is prototyping. Aim of this phase is to choose an idea that seems to be suitable for your purposes and start to work on it further. Prototyping makes the ideas into a concrete representation. Prototype is a physical representation of an idea or solution, that is easy to create and gives you test ideas at low fidelity and cost. Low-fidelity prototyping is an optimal way to create a representation of your ideas to be tested. In this way you can rapidly try and test many rough ideas. Prototyping gives you the opportunity to make your ideas into a tangible format to be tested among the end-users [19, 21].

The fifth phase of the design thinking process is testing. Aim of this phase is to test the complete product and service using the best solutions identified during the prototyping phase. This phase is an iterative process; the results generated during the testing phase are often used to refine one or more problems and understand users, the conditions of use, how people think, behave, and feel. Goal is to understand the product or service and its users as well possible. When the testing takes place in a real situation in real environment of the end-users, the more valuable information the session of testing will bring to the designer. At its best you get a grasp of how people understand, perceive, and accept your idea by just observing them when using and experiencing the prototype [2, 4, 12].

Even the phases are described in a numerical order, the process of design thinking is not linear itself, merely iterative (Fig. 1.1). The learning curve the process offers for the designers and developers, is fruitful and insightful and usually gives

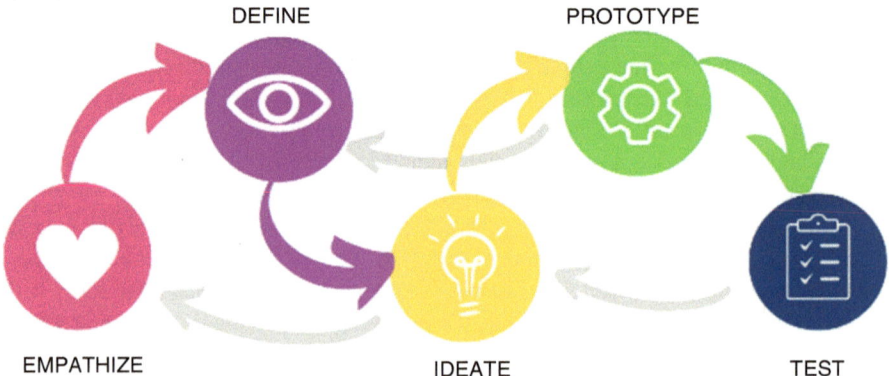

Fig. 1.1 Design thinking process

the designers and developers the possibility but also forces them to go back to previous phase(s) to learn more from the users, to redefine the problem, or to alleviate the pitfalls which may occur during prototyping and testing. Therefore, design thinking approach may be the key to gain more effective, attractive, feasible, and sustainable solutions for healthcare [4, 13].

Even though design thinking process we provide herein ends to the testing phase, there is work after that. The whole implementation process needs also time and effort, before the solutions designed and developed can be real part of the healthcare. Sometimes the innovations coming from the design thinking loop are such that they should be commercialized. This demands a whole new process of doing. Chapter 8 talks about business models and offers commercialization scenarios.

1.4   Healthcare Needs Ways to Address Its Challenges

Aging population, complex health challenges, financial pressures, shortage of healthcare staff, and the demand for patient-centered approach in healthcare provide the basis for applying design thinking to develop better healthcare services and health technology solutions.

The aging population and the growing need for care is a global phenomenon. At the same time, the health problems of the population are becoming increasingly complex and require a wide range of expertise, the ability to work together in a multidisciplinary way and services that enable us to provide quality care to clients and patients. Moreover, the rising cost of healthcare and the increasing number of patients being treated will not bring relief, but rather challenge providers to develop financially sustainable ways to ensure the sustainability of healthcare [22, 23].

With increasing numbers of clients and patients, the risk of a shortage of care is high. This situation is not helped by the current trend of health workers moving to other sectors, which can be seen in many countries. Healthcare jobs are not attractive, and there are fewer and fewer young people to choose this field as a future career. The shortage of healthcare staff is becoming one of the most demanding tasks to solve in healthcare in future. Global challenges such as pandemics are highlighting many shortcomings in the health sector, such as staff fatigue, inefficient supply chains, and insufficient adaptability of services. This does little to make healthcare an attractive and compelling field [24].

Modern healthcare calls for patient-centered care and services [7, 8]. New products and services, especially those based on digitalization, offer a better opportunity to deliver personalized care than before. However, it is not always self-evident that care and services can be provided equally to all patients. The development of products and services should therefore consider not only the needs and views of end-users but also the ethical values of healthcare. Design thinking focuses on the needs and perspectives of the individual. It provides a good model for patient-centeredness in the design of products and services [4, 7–9]. Chapter 2 focuses on design thinking and innovations in healthcare from the ethical perspective.

There is therefore a clear need to deliver solutions that will help us meet these challenges in the future. High-quality products and services may free up staff for other tasks and make healthcare more attractive. Through innovation we can solve many of the challenges in healthcare. Implementing design thinking methods, we offer the healthcare staff a greater involvement for the design and development. When their skills, knowledge, and expertise are valued, it may increase their professional pride and yet help with the shortcomings of the staff. People matter, which is the essence of design thinking. Collaboration and working together gives a new mindset to working and increases the capacity for interdisciplinary working. At the best utilization of design thinking approach in healthcare, we have the ability to deliver adaptive and agile solutions to solve the challenges. Chapter 6 talks about the use of design thinking in the day-to-day management and leadership in nursing.

1.5   Design Thinking Can Support Healthcare Staff to Innovate

The opportunity of healthcare staff to detect challenges and problems in healthcare is huge. Day-to-day operation in the hospitals and other health institutions makes staff one of the best experts on the current development needs. Healthcare staff, in other words, may also act as innovators, designers, and developers. Design thinking offers professionals with an optimal structure, steps, and framework which can be used when designing and developing new products and services to healthcare [11, 13, 14]. There is also importance of providing the staff with education on using and implementing design thinking tools and methods. Continuing education possibilities offer the staff with the opportunity to learn design thinking. Chapter 4 talks about design thinking in healthcare education.

Research on the use of design thinking in healthcare is evolving. There is nowadays more and more of evidence on its potential and success in healthcare. Design thinking interventions have showed greater satisfaction, usability, and effectiveness [13]. Implementation of design thinking approaches within healthcare can help drive necessary innovation in care processes [4]. Design thinking can be used to address challenges in a variety of domains related to the patient experience [9]. Design thinking is widely applicable in healthcare to all actions involving disease prevention and treatment [25]. More evidence on the use of design thinking in healthcare is described in the Chap. 5.

References

1. Braha D, Reich Y (2003) Topological structures for modeling engineering design processes. Res Eng Des 14(4):185–199. https://doi.org/10.1007/s00163-003-0035-3
2. Razzouk R, Shute V (2012) What is design thinking and why is it important? Rev Educ Res 82(3):330–348. https://doi.org/10.3102/0034654312457429
3. Maula H, Maula J (2019) Design ja johtaminen. Alma Talent, Helsinki
4. Roberts JP, Fisher TR, Trowbridge MJ, Bent C (2016) A design thinking framework for healthcare management and innovation. Healthc (Amst) 4(1):11–14. https://doi.org/10.1016/j.hjdsi.2015.12.002

5. Bernstein A (2015) The evolution of design thinking (full issue). Harvard Business Review, September, p 93
6. McLaughlin JE, Wolcott MD, Hubbard D, Umstead K, Rider TR (2019) A qualitative review of the design thinking framework in health professions education. BMC Med Educ 19(1):98. https://doi.org/10.1186/s12909-019-1528-8
7. Epstein RM, Fiscella K, Lesser CS, Stange KC (2010) Why the nation needs a policy push on patient-centered health care. Health Aff (Millwood) 29(8):1489–1495. https://doi.org/10.1377/hlthaff.2009.0888
8. Cliff B (2012) The evolution of patient-centered care. J Healthc Manag 57(2):86–88. https://doi.org/10.1097/00115514-201203000-00003
9. Kim SH, Myers CG, Allen L (2017) Health care providers can use design thinking to improve patient experiences. Harv Bus Rev 95(5):222–229
10. Dell'Era C, Magistretti S, Cautela C, Verganti R, Zurlo F (2020) Four kinds of design thinking: from ideating to making, engaging, and criticizing. Creat Innov Manag 29(2):324–344. https://doi.org/10.1111/caim.12353
11. Austin C (2015) Design thinking: expanding the frame of reference. A study of concepts, ideas and thinking tools developed by Edward de Bono that have potential within a design process and design thinking framework. Doctor of Philosophy Thesis, Swinburne University. https://researchbank.swinburne.edu.au/items/a3edaa30-f026-4992-af96-1fb05c8ccc3e/1/
12. Waidelich L, Richter A, Kolmel B, Bulander R (2018) Design thinking process model review. In: 2018 IEEE international conference on engineering, technology and innovation (ICE/ITMC). IEEE, Cardiff
13. Altman M, Huang TTK, Breland JY (2018) Design thinking in health care. Prev Chronic Dis 15(180128):E117. https://doi.org/10.5888/pcd15.180128
14. Badwan B, Bothara R, Latijnhouwers M, Smithies A, Sandars J (2018) The importance of design thinking in medical education. Med Teach 40(4):425–426. https://doi.org/10.1080/0142159X.2017.1399203
15. Martin RL (2009) The opposable mind: winning through integrative thinking. Harvard Business Press, Boston
16. Plattner H, Meinel C (2010) In: Leifer L (ed) Design thinking: understand-improve-apply. Springer Science & Business Media, Berlin
17. Geissdoerfer M, Bocken NMP, Hultink EJ (2016) Design thinking to enhance the sustainable business modelling process – a workshop based on a value mapping process. J Clean Prod 135:1218–1232. https://doi.org/10.1016/j.jclepro.2016.07.020
18. Cross N (2001) Designerly ways of knowing: design discipline versus design science. Des Issues 17(3):49–55. https://doi.org/10.1162/074793601750357196
19. Oliveira M, Zancul E, Fleury AL (2021) Design thinking as an approach for innovation in healthcare: systematic review and research avenues. BMJ Innov 7(2):491–498. https://doi.org/10.1136/bmjinnov-2020-000428
20. Stempfle J, Badke-Schaube P (2002) Thinking in design teams-an analysis of team communication. Des Stud 23:473–496
21. Seidel VP, Fixson SK (2013) Adopting design thinking in novice multidisciplinary teams: the application and limits of design methods and reflexive practices: adopting design thinking in novice teams. J Prod Innov Manag 30:19–33. https://doi.org/10.1111/jpim.12061
22. Ogura S, Jakovljevic MM (2018) Global population aging-health care, social and economic consequences. Front Public Health 6:335
23. Feng Z (2019) Global convergence: aging and long-term care policy challenges in the developing world. J Aging Soc Policy 31(4):291–297. https://doi.org/10.1080/08959420.2019.1626205
24. World Health Organization (2016) Global strategy on human resources for health: workforce 2030. WHO document production services, Geneva; Available from: https://apps.who.int/iris/bitstream/handle/10665/250368/?sequence=1
25. Ferreira FK, Song EH, Gomes H, Garcia EB, Ferreira LM (2015) New mindset in scientific method in the health field: design thinking. Clinics (Sao Paulo) 70(12):770–772. https://doi.org/10.6061/clinics/2015(12)01

Ethical Aspects and Innovations in Healthcare

Helena Siipi and Mari Kangasniemi

2.1 Introduction

Ethical analysis is much needed in healthcare innovation context for various reasons. First, the necessity for the analysis grows from fundamental purpose of the healthcare which is both practical and ethical by nature. From practical point of view, the purpose of healthcare is to provide services on the most effective, efficient, and economical way to get and maintain inhabitants' health and well-being with limited resources. This requires constant development of services and processes, including innovation development. From ethical point of view, the same target can be seen as to enable best possible care and service for biggest possible amount of service users. In addition, health and well-being as the targets of healthcare can be understood as intrinsically valuable: They are good, right, and fundaments of life for any human individual, and the aim of healthcare services is to promote and support them. As a result, also the targets and processes through which the healthcare innovations are developed and used are under special attention: what kind of impact they have on well-being, health and life of individuals and groups. This means that balancing between practical and ethical values is a part of design thinking. The question is how aware the researchers and developers are of it.

Second, ethical reflection on design thinking [1] in healthcare is always multidimensional. There are numerous stakeholders and interests involved in the medical

H. Siipi
Department of Philosophy, Contemporary History and Political Science, University of Turku, Turku, Finland
e-mail: helsii@utu.fi

M. Kangasniemi (✉)
Faculty of Medicine, Department of Nursing Science, University of Turku, Turku, Finland

Satakunta Wellbeing Services County, Turku, Finland
e-mail: mari.kangasniemi@utu.fi

© The Author(s), under exclusive license to Springer Nature
Switzerland AG 2023
A. Pakarinen et al. (eds.), *Design Thinking in Healthcare*,
https://doi.org/10.1007/978-3-031-24510-7_2

field from individuals such as patients and their families to professionals, private and public service providers, companies, and researchers. They represent different disciplines, world views, and cultural and religious values. Making their different interest visible increases ethical awareness in the innovation process. Yet, this may not always be simple as power relationships subsist within and between the different interest groups. In addition, the stakeholder groups are usually somehow excluding, rising a question how minority and other vulnerable groups are recognized.

2.2   Empathy as Ethical Concept

2.2.1   Empathy as a Part of Design Thinking Process

The first phase of design thinking process, empathy or empathizing, refers to the responsiveness to experiences to the views of the stakeholders [2, 3]. It can be seen as a factor that designates design thinking from other ways of creation [4]. Empathy is seen central as it enables the designers to understand the needs and challenges of the stakeholders which, in turn, will be integral for finding new and innovative solutions that are suitable for them [4, 5].

The fact that design thinking process starts from empathizing is interesting and quite revolutionary. In western thought, rationality has tended to be the method for decision-making. The interest in empathizing has raised from acknowledging the dangers of rationalism: Rationalism "may facilitate us to ignore the lived experiences of others and replace the subjectivity and individual worth of those others with utilitarian calculations" [5, 6]. At its best, the human ability to empathize can allow a designer to understand what are the members of the relevant stakeholder group going through, learn from them, and take their view into account in the innovation work [2, 5].

2.2.2   What Does Empathy Mean?

From ethical point of view, the process of design thinking can be ethically sound only if empathy can form an ethical basis for an innovation process. The role of empathy in moral behavior (including innovation) has been studied to some extent in last few years with very differing outcomes. Paul Bloom (2016) [1], for example, is against it whereas Slote [7] sees all morality to be based on empathy. In what follows we will argue that using empathy as a starting point requires ethical awareness regarding certain issues. Some of these issues to be discussed are especially important in the context of healthcare and, thus, call for attention when applying design thinking to healthcare.

As a concept, empathy refers to ability to place oneself into a position of another. In so-called projective empathy we put ourselves into the situation of another and imagine what we ourselves would feel in their place. The so-called simulative empathy is more other-directed and instead of asking, what would I feel in their place, I ask what the other feels in their situation [6]. In design thinking, projective empathy is not sufficient for good innovation work as it may leave the other person unnoticed. What a patient with schizophrenia, for example, feels in hospital, may be totally different to what a more mentally well-being person would feel at the same hospital environment. Thus, the design thinking relies on simulative empathy (see, e.g., descriptions of empathizing in design thinking [1, 2, 5]). In practice, this need to adapt to the others' point of view usually requires direct data collection or interviewing among target group. However, it is important also to understand the limits of simulative empathy. The human beings do not have direct access to minds of others and, thus, simulative empathy is always somehow non-perfect and prone to misunderstandings.

In design thinking it might be useful to acknowledge different varieties of empathy. Empathy has various varieties and they all do not equally support morality [1, 6]. Thus, ethical soundness of the innovation process and outcome may depend on variety of empathy adopted to design thinking.

So-called cognitive empathy is about human ability to notice—either by direct perceiving or by inferring—the emotive states of others [6]. In cognitive empathy we note the other and rationally conclude their feelings and emotions from facial expressions, tone of voice, ways of behavior, and other clues. Aaltola (2018, p. 58) [6] describes cognitive empathy to be an emotionally cool or neutral state. It allows us to understand others but does not in itself include emotions. The challenge of cognitive empathy is that it is really an interpretation. The feelings and emotions of other persons are detected from their behavior and, as with any interpretation, there is a possibility of making mistakes. Thus, if this type of empathy is used as a starting point of design thinking, one needs to be aware of this possibility and limits of one's capacities. Yet, of course, with the needed awareness it is a valuable tool.

Contrary to cognitive empathy, affective empathy includes emotional responding to affective states of others. Affective empathy is intrinsically involved and includes going with the feeling of another person. It is often fast, almost automatic response. When we see someone to hit his thump with a hammer, we instantly feel his pain [6]. The problem with affective empathy is that the knowledge gained through it is always limited—at least in the complex world. People do always openly show their affective states and they may even purposefully mislead other regarding them. As Aaltola (2018, p. 87) [6] puts it, "both cognitive and affective empathy are required for the type of understanding of others that dwells deeper than obvious."

The reflective empathy consists of understanding the emotions of another person—either just by perceiving them or also by going with the affection. However, in reflective empathy the emotions of another person are not just let to guide the contents of the empathy but rather the observer intentionally reflects on them. In other words, we give "attention to what we know of or feel with another and what sort of mental contents of our own impact our judgement or experience. In short, we empathize and then adopt a metaperspective into the process of empathy" [6]. According to Aaltola (2018, pp. 132–133) [6] in reflective empathy we move back and forth between empathy and the metalevel and that will give us clear perception of the situation as well as experience of the other as well as of our own responses. In that way, reflective empathy gives a picture about with whom, why, and on what grounds we empathize. Moreover, it gives us understanding about limitations of the empathizing process. It is important to notice that reflective empathy is not just theoretical possibility, it is a human skill, and we all use it sometimes. It is also a skill that can be developed and cultivated.

2.2.3 Who Will Be Empathized?

The crucial question for the ethics of design thinking is, who the designers will empathize? Empathy is always empathy toward someone. The guides for design thinking usually highlight not just the importance of hearing the experts, but also engaging the individuals from different stakeholder groups who will be either use or otherwise affected by the innovation to be developed. The goal is to deeply understand their insights, needs, and challenges regarding the issue involved [4]. Thus, the ethically critical issue concerns selection of the relevant stakeholder groups, as well as individuals, who will represent their group in the innovation process.

But who are the relevant stakeholders? The question is important regarding all design thinking but ethically exceptionally serious regarding the context of healthcare. There some individuals and groups are in a vulnerable position and where problems in usability of innovations may turn out to have devastating consequences. The relevant stakeholders include, obviously, patients and clients as well as healthcare professionals. Yet, experiences of different patients may differ considerably and, thus, choice of their representatives may greatly influence the outcome. Should, for example, one involve long-term patients or the ones with new diagnosis, patient organization activists, or ones randomly selected from the healthcare unit? Further questions concern inclusion of other stakeholders. Family members and close ones seem to inherently important, for example, in development of innovations for the neonatal care units. However, it is also important to notice that views, experiences, and feelings of the clients may differ from those of their family members, for example, regarding elderly care and housing for disabled. In some cases, for example, regarding severely autistic clients, empathizing requires professional expertise (e.g., regarding communication). Not just who is accepted as a relevant stakeholder but also who is left out is ethically important. Should, for example, individuals refusing the treatment or the ones who do not have access to care be included in the process?

These questions become obvious, for example, when considering design thinking regarding palliative care. On the one hand, palliative care could certainly benefit from new innovations and it is obvious that the experiences of patients are central to their development. On the other hand, the above-presented problems regarding inclusion and exclusion are easy to see. Most of the dying patients and their close ones probably do not have strength to participate in design thinking processes. Those how can participate may not be representative group. Most importantly, palliative care is often under-resourced and not all patients who need it get it. As a result, clients of palliative care units have already been selected as all dying patients do not have equal access to this type of care [8]. Thus, including only clients from palliative care units might distort the empathizing process as it misses the voices of those who do not reach the care they need. The example shows, in short, that since design thinking rests so heavily on the stage of empathizing—it is the starting point for the whole process—and since the questions of inclusion are central to ethics of healthcare, applying design thinking to healthcare requires careful and ethically sensitive planning regarding whom the developers will be empathizing.

2.2.4   Can We Empathize Justly and Equally?

More problems arise from the fact that our empathy reflects our biases: It is easier to feel empathy toward individuals who are familiar and socially close to us, who are similar to us, and who we see as attractive or vulnerable. Positive experiences with someone increase empathy toward his or her, whereas seeing someone as scary decreases empathy [1, 6]. Most importantly, this kind of bias is often implicit. The implicit biases are not acknowledged by us, and they may be contrary to our conscious thoughts and values. Thus, even if a designer intellectually believes that suffering of members of different ethnic groups, age groups, sexual orientation groups, socio-economic groups and lifestyle groups, for example, is equally serious, the designer still tends to feel most empathy toward individuals who are similar to her. Implicit biases are common, and they have strong influence on our behavior. Healthcare professionals exhibit the same level of implicit biases than wider population [1, 9].

This problem of implicit biases will probably be most serious in situations where stakeholders have conflicting views or interests—that is when the situation is such that designer cannot simultaneously satisfy desires, needs, and wants of all different stakeholders [10]. In the reality of sometimes poorly resourced public healthcare, such situation may not be uncommon. Thus, there is a danger that basing the design process in empathy leads into favoring members of some groups on the expense of groups that are more foreign to the designer. This is an ethically serious outcome and should be somehow tackled in the design thinking process. In the minimum, the designers should become aware of their biases.

2.2.5   Limits of Empathy in Design Thinking

Empathy-based decision-making has further challenges. The problems arise from the same source as the strength of empathy—that is from its focus on individuals' needs, challenges, and viewpoints. Since empathy focuses on specific individuals and their lived experiences, it is insensitive to statistical data and cost-benefit analyses. Thus, it may lead into ignoring the effects our decisions have on groups of people—an outcome that cannot be irrelevant to healthcare-related decision-making [1]. This will be highlighted by the following example:

Imagine learning that a faulty vaccine has caused Rebecca Smith, an adorable eight-year-old, to get extremely sick. If you watch her suffering and listen to her and her family, the empathy will flow, and you'll want to act. But suppose that stopping the vaccine program will cause, say, a dozen random children to die. Here your empathy is silent—how can you empathize with statistical abstraction [1]?

Thus, it seems obvious that in order to be ethically sound, the design thinking process cannot rest solely on the empathy. In the context of healthcare especially that might lead into ethically very bad decisions. Thus, the understanding gained through the empathizing needs in design thinking to be somehow fit together and balanced with the evidence-based nursing and medicine practices. In addition, and especially in public healthcare, one also needs to acknowledge the limited resources. (Yet, at its best, design thinking may contribute to more efficient use of those resources.)

2.3   Problem Defining and Risk for Medicalization

As the aim of design thinking in healthcare is to create new products, treatments, devices, services, or processes, and from ethical point of view, design thinking crosses the question of medicalization. As a concept, medicalization refers to the process where problems which were not taken to be medical become to be treated as medical. According to the classical and still widely used [11] definition by Conrad [12], "medicalization consists of defining a problem in medical terms, using medical language to describe a problem, adopting a medical framework to understand a problem, or using a medical intervention to 'treat' it." Thus, not only biomedical knowledge but many different forms of medical knowledge can medicalize aspects of life [13]. That has been accelerated by advanced technology, producing new or more expanded or sophisticated knowledge of life. Medicalization as a concept can be extended to the health problematization, where the health needs will be produced regarding issues which originally did not require intervention. The consequence is that producing new means for solving health problems will provoke new health needs, wishes, and expectations. In addition, medicalization [14] has predicted to cause over-treatment and over-use of services.

Design thinking can be related also to the distinction between the scope of praxis and the aim of praxis by Correia (2017) [12]. He has described that as the scope of praxis, medical decisions are intrinsically context dependent. However, as the "aim of the practice, while the categories 'health' and 'disease' have changed drastically, the aim of medicine can be identified as the quest for ordered explanations and intervention aimed at treatment or healing." Thus, within the aim of practice design thinking may seek for interventions or means to promote health or alleviate suffering or managing of diseases.

It is noteworthy that the medicalization does not only take place through the medical interest. It is increasingly through the efforts of patients and citizens who are seeking to legitimize their distress through defining it as a "medical" problem (Correia 2017) where they are not as passive stakeholders in medicalization [15]. Then the increased concerns over risk and a decline in the trust of expert authority led to the situation where "the modern day 'consumer' of healthcare plays an active role in bringing about or resisting medicalization." Thus, the modern-day consumer requires consideration of the specific social context in which medicalization occurs [16]. Currently, the ideology of eternal health and life may cause pressures to endless seek for means to achieve health and well-being. This causes inequity and polarization but also costs for individual patients and clients. Thus, with regard to design thinking, the understanding what the scope of the product is and how it is related to the concept of health is needed. What kind of health and well-being concept it represents?

Medicalization has also seen as a part of health promotion: early detection of symptoms and health problems has seen as attractive for patients and healthcare staff. In addition to primary, secondary, and tertiary prevention, a quaternary prevention has linkage to medicalization [17]. It has referred to "action taken to identify patient at risk of overmedicalization, to protect him from new medical invasion, and to suggest to him interventions, which are ethically acceptable" [18]. Thus, on the design thinking, it is needed to consider, what kind of orientation of health promotion they have. For healthcare it can sometimes be a strategy for improving population health and well-being. On the design thinking process, the analysis of the scope of healthcare and medicine will make visible their relationship. What is the acceptable target and how the innovation is related to the aim and scope of healthcare and medicine. It is connected to the promises for patients and clients.

2.4 Sustainable Development and Design Thinking

2.4.1 Dimensions of Sustainability

An inherent starting point for design thinking is to provide new innovations that are suitable to target group or purpose [5]. The process can be carried out by using diverse materials to produce various commodities.

Sustainable development can be defined as "development that meets the needs of the present without compromising the ability of future generations to meet their own needs" described in the UN sustainable development goals 2022 [19]. United Nation (2022) [20] has defined 17 different sustainable development goals which are urgent call for action by all countries in a global partnership. Sustainable development can be organized on four main dimensions which are social, cultural, economic, and environmental dimensions [21]. The heart of sustainable development is the concern regarding future generations: The needs of the present people should be fulfilled but in ways that do not compromise the chances of future generations to meet their own needs [22].

In the context of design thinking, the social and cultural dimensions of sustainability highlight the question of how the innovation is related to the surrounding society and era. Socially sustainable innovations simultaneously benefit society and enable people to maintain diversity of cultural values, practices, and chains from heritage to the future [23]. According to UN (2022) [19, 20] companies have both direct and indirect effects for employees, workers, customers, and local communities. In the similar way, innovation by design thinking may potentially affect large number of people. All those effects should be acknowledged in socially and culturally sustainable innovation. The special attention is on the human rights and equality of specific groups such as women, children, and people with disabilities. In short, the focus is on how innovation work can contribute on the lives of the people it affects, creating goods and services that help them meet basic needs and more inclusive value chain.

The economic sustainability refers to use and maintenance of resources in a way that they will create long-term sustainable values by optimal use, recovery, and recycling [24]. Regarding the design thinking in healthcare this implies that one needs to consider not only the straight cost of the development process but also what the produced innovation will cost in the healthcare system in future. On these calculations, it needs to be recognized, first, how the product will replace some current practices and what is their cost-relationship, and second, whether the product is a complementary product for existing services and what type of new costs it will cause. Third, on need to take into account what kind of new needs the product will cause and whether may it increase the use of services in short- or long-term period in future.

The first three dimensions of sustainable development are anthropocentric as the focus is in the present and future humans. The fourth dimension, environmental sustainability can be interpreted in anthropocentric or biocentric way. According to the anthropocentric understanding, nature and environment are resources which should be used wisely so that the future generations will also have access to them. Nature is certainly seen valuable—but first and foremost instrumentally valuable [22]. This kind of sustainability requirement is about preserving an environment that is healthy and habitable for present and future humans [25].

The biocentric interpretation of environmental sustainability is called ecological sustainability. Ecological sustainability highlights the importance of living in ways that enable the continuation of the healthy living planet and biosphere. The interest is not solely on needs of present and future humans but also on present and future members of other species, ecosystems, and the life-supporting system on earth in general [25, 26]. In order to meet the requirements of ecological sustainability, the design thinking process should have means for including environmental concerns in this broad sense. Ecological sustainability is a challenge for the design thinking-based innovation as it is obvious that the plants, animals, and ecosystems—let alone the biosphere—will not have their direct representatives on the stakeholder groups.

2.4.2 Sustainability on Design Thinking

The challenges sustainable development set for the design thinking have been acknowledged by various authors and many of them have contributed into developing design thinking models that integrate sustainability targets to its process [21, 27, 28]. These models highlight the necessity of spelling out what sustainability is understood to mean on that particular innovation process as well as forming clear criteria for succeeding in sustainable innovation [28]. In practice, this requires throughout and careful contemplation on environmentally sufficient and, yet, feasible goals.

The innovations made today influence present stakeholders but also future human beings [27]. Thus, the challenge for the design thinking is interesting and clear: How to include the interests of the future people into the process? Design thinking process does not automatically incorporate the needs of future generations [28]. This is not a surprise as design thinking is centered to present stakeholder experiences and, in this sense, prioritizes immediate users [21, 27]. For Hoolohan and Brownie [27], this is a challenging limitation. There is a danger that the future people and their interests will be left unnoticed. According to Shapira et al. [28, p. 281] sustainability is usually included in the design thinking process only if the designer wants to incorporate it as a personal value. They further rise a worry that as design thinking concentrates on the desires and experiences of the stakeholders it may contribute to developing products and services which (unintentionally) continue or strengthen current course of unsustainable lifestyle [28]. This all is true also about the healthcare context. Innovations developed for healthcare today will have major impacts for the lives of future people. Thus, in the name of sustainable development, their needs should be somehow acknowledged in the innovation process.

The challenge with goals is to balance between feasibility and what is sufficient from the environmental point of view. That climate change requires considerable lifestyle changes is known by everybody. Yet, at the same time, goals should be reachable and realistic. Birkeland [26, p. 164], for example, sets a high standard for sustainability in stating that an innovation cannot be sustainable if the life support system would be better off without it. How this should be understood regarding innovations which replace older and more polluting technologies but still cause harm to the environment? Certainly, not every small improvement is sufficient for an innovation to be sustainable. On the other side of the coin, in practice, carbon neutrality is seldom possible.

The further challenge for innovation in healthcare (which may be shared by various other fields as well) is the multitude of connections between healthcare and climate change. Climate change causes health problems and, thus, also increases the burden of healthcare services. Yet, at the same time, healthcare system is a source of emissions. According to Pichler et al. [29, p. 1] healthcare on average accounts 5% of national Co_2 footprint at OECD countries. Thus, conflicts between sustainability goals and human health and well-being goals can take place: as a simple example, usage of disposable tools for hygiene reasons may not nicely fit together with sustainability goals. Moreover, even though the stakeholders may (some of them may not) sympathize the sustainability goals, they may still be hesitant to compromise the fulfillment of their desires and wants. Thus, including the sustainability goals into design thinking process may lead into hard dilemmas to be solved [21].

On the other side of coin, sustainability-integrated design thinking and its creative optimist approach may also be valuable tool for solving conflicts between sustainability goals and stakeholder needs. Combining the complete understanding of the stakeholders' experiences with well-defined sustainability goals may at its best enhance new innovative solutions which enable fitting together goals that at first seemed contradictory. Thus, sustainability-aware and enriched design thinking may well serve not just the needs of stakeholders but also sustainability goals [26, 28]. At its best, design thinking can be taken as an opportunity that has potential to influence healthcare services and increase the inclusion of sustainability targets to healthcare innovation and decision-making. This, however, cannot be expected to happen automatically or by itself but only after conscious and careful inclusion of the sustainability aspects to the design thinking process. Shapira et al. [28, p. 284] recommend integrating the selected sustainability goals to all parts of the innovation process, possibly as numerous small add-ins.

2.5   Research Ethics in Innovations

Depending on the approach, design thinking in healthcare can be identified as research or developmental work of product or service. The principal characteristic of research is to produce new knowledge and the principal characteristic of developmental work is to produce improved practices. Despite to their differences, the intention of both research and developmental work is to produce new ideas or approaches and, thus, they always are value based. Thus, in line with other research and developmental work in healthcare, also the design thinking process is guided by ethical principles of biomedical research [30] and codes of conduct [31]. The primary aim of principles of biomedical ethics is to protect human subjects in the study and guide researchers to carry out research without intended or unintended harm for participants in the study [30, 31]. Design thinking is very human centered. Participation of human subjects of stakeholder groups is integral for the process and human subjects are also the final user of the product or service. It is noteworthy how privacy, autonomy, equity, and informed consent have been ensured during the innovation process [32].

2.5.1   Justification of Innovations

From research ethics point of view, the fundamental question in design thinking is the justification of innovation because the characteristic of innovation cannot simply presuppose that innovation is "inherently good" [33]. Justification refers to consideration of the needs for innovation, the characteristics of innovation itself, and the impact of innovation [32]. However, justification of needs, characteristics, and impact of innovations differ depending on the point of views of different stakeholders and their values. The needs for innovations may, among other things, be based on climate change, resource depletion, poverty alleviation, or aging societies [34]. Decision makers, innovators, or clients may have different approaches, and they can imply an ethical dilemma between different stakeholders [32]. Technological innovation processes have traditionally been based on commercialization of innovative products and services. In addition to economic values, innovations can also be

Table 2.1 The value domains and dimensions of responsible innovation in health [35]

Value domain	Dimension
Population health	Health relevance: does the innovation address a relevant health problem? Ethical, legal, and social issues: was the innovation developed by seeking to mitigate its ethical, legal, and social issues? Health equity: in what ways the innovation promotes health equity?
Health system	Inclusiveness: were the innovation development inclusive? Responsiveness: does the innovation provide a dynamic solution to a health system need or challenge? Level of care: is the level of care required by the innovation compatible with health system sustainability?
Economic	Frugality: does the innovation deliver greater value to more people using fewer resources?
Organizational	Business model: does the organization that produces the innovation seek to provide more value to user, purchases, and society?
Environmental	Eco-responsibility: does the innovation limits its negative environmental impacts throughout its lifecycle as much possible?

motivated on the benefits to users through products and services in terms of ease of use, functionality, efficiency, and novelty. It is noteworthy that innovations can also have undesirable consequences for society and environment. In healthcare context the critical problems are the unpredictability and uncertainty of those negative ethical impacts [32].

As noted above, different stakeholders from micro to macro level [32] may have different value domains on innovations in health. According to Pacifico Silva et al. [35], these domains can be divided on population health, health system, economic, organizational, and environmental levels (Table 2.1). Justification of innovation requires rethinking what we want from innovation and what kind of future we want innovation to bring into healthcare [36].

2.5.2 Responsibilities of Different Stakeholders

The second question concerns roles and responsibilities of different stakeholders on innovation process (Table 2.2). Roles, responsibilities, and ethical concerns vary among various stakeholders [32] from director-level responsibilities to facilitate financing to government and policy-makers responsibilities to enable conditions for innovation development to achieve well-being of citizens. Also, funders have a crucial role in directing innovations [36]. In addition, scientists, universities [36], and researchers have a central role. The primary role of researchers is to provide new knowledge or improved practices, and they have intellectual property rights for them. According to research ethics, their primary responsibility is to protect research subjects and to avoid and decrease harm for them. This is also a question in the innovation process: beyond the innovation itself, the focus is on the participants and research integrity.

Table 2.2 Stakeholder mapping [32] modified in design thinking in healthcare

Stakeholders	Type	Interests	Rights	Responsibilities/ duties	Ethical concerns/ dilemmas
Directors	Dominant	Finance performance of the firm: bonus, payments, power, prestige	Make decisions in the interests of stakeholders	Fiduciary; legal compliance	Moral hazard; product safety
Customers/ patients	Dependent	Products and services at affordable price with quality	Product safety; fair price; good information; privacy	Product usage according to the intended usage and procedure	Safety; equity in terms of affordability and accessibility; efficacy; data protection
Media	Demanding	Newsworthy publication, usually bad press	Freedom of information	Accuracy of information; timely information	Accessibility; variability of information
Government	Dominant	Well-being of the citizens	Corporate tax	Protect citizens and the public environment	Public interests
Researchers[a]	Dominant	Provide new knowledge or improved practices	Intellectual property rights	Protect research subjects	Avoiding and decreasing harm for research subjects, research integrity
Designers[a]	Dominant	Provide new tools, equipment or practices; commercial interests	Intellectual property rights	Safety and ethics in design thinking	Commercial interests

[a]Added in this chapter

The question is, what is the role of innovator in design thinking? If the role of innovators has been considered as researchers, the protection of research subject as a main principle of research ethics is guiding their role. However, the goal of innovation is often focused on providing new tools, equipment, and practices and targeted to commercial goals. Thus, the roles of innovator and researcher might have different, sometimes contractionary interests and cause ethical dilemmas for working. Awareness of different roles, interest, and ethical rights and responsibilities may support stakeholders to identify ethics in design thinking process.

2.6   Conclusions

A good ethical analysis is necessarily multidimensional as it needs to acknowledge various ethically relevant factors. The ethically relevant factors concern rights and needs of individuals involved. At the same time, a good ethical analysis takes into consideration those social, economic, ecological, and cultural aspects which influence the ethical acceptability of innovations. Ideally innovations are just, efficient, low-cost, environment friendly, and responsive to different lifestyles and world views. In practice, the different ethically relevant factors do not always point toward the same direction. Maximizing patient autonomy, for example, may in some cases conflict with ecological sustainability. In similar lines, efficiency may sometimes compromise privacy or some other patient right. Thus, the ethical analysis often consists of balancing different ethically relevant factors against each other to form the ethically acceptable and sustainable solution.

The big question is whether the process of innovation is sufficient for exposing all factors that should, from the ethical point of view, be acknowledged in an ethically excellent innovation process. Especially, how can one make empathizing (and design thinking in general) sensitive enough regarding environmental concerns, necessity of climate actions, and needs of future generations? In short, given the seriousness of the climate change and other environmental crises, all innovation work should acknowledge the sustainability requirements. On what conditions can design thinking do so?

A responsible research-based innovation process is a transparent, interactive process by which societal actors and innovators become mutually responsive to each other with a view to the (ethical) acceptability, sustainability, and societal desirability of the innovation process and its products (to allow a proper embedding of scientific and technological advances in our society) [37]. Thus, responsible innovation process requires a circular reflection with embedded ethical decision-making [32]. At its best, incorporating ethical principles in the design process does not only serve ethics but can lead to well-accepted technological advances [37]. In order to achieve multidimensional ethical analysis on design thinking process, attention needs to be paid on researchers' and innovators' ethical awareness, willingness to include ethics on all stages of the design process, and educational support for succeeding in this.

References

1. Bloom P (2016) Against empathy: the case for rational compassion. Ecco. ISBN 978-0-06-233935-5
2. Hamington M (2019) Integrating care ethics and design thinking. J Bus Ethics 155(1):91–103. https://doi.org/10.1007/s10551-017-3522-6
3. Buchanan R (1992) Wicked problems in design thinking. Des Issues 8(2):5. https://doi.org/10.2307/1511637
4. Maula H, Maula J (2019) Design ja johtaminen. Alma Talent, Helsinki
5. Mcdonagh D, Thomas J (2010) Rethinking design thinking: empathy supporting innovation. Australas Med J 1(3):458–464

6. Aaltola E (2018) Varieties of empathy: moral psychology and animal ethics. Rowman & Littlefield International, London
7. Slote M (2007) The ethics of care and empathy. Routledge, New York
8. de Veer AJE, Stringer B, van Meijel B, Verkaik R, Francke AL (2018) Access to palliative care for homeless people: complex lives, complex care. BMC Palliat Care 17(1):119. https://doi.org/10.1186/s12904-018-0368-3
9. FitzGerald C, Hurst S (2017) Implicit bias in healthcare professionals: a systematic review. BMC Med Ethics 18(1):19. https://doi.org/10.1186/s12910-017-0179-8
10. Dorst K (2011) The core of 'design thinking' and its application. Des Stud 32(6):521–532. https://doi.org/10.1016/j.destud.2011.07.006
11. van Dijk W, Meinders MJ, Tanke MA, Westert GP, Jeurissen PP (2020) Medicalization defined in empirical contexts – A scoping review. International journal of health policy and management 9(8): 327–334. https://doi.org/10.15171/ijhpm.2019.101
12. Conrad P (1992) Medicalization and social control. Annu Rev Sociol 18(1):209–232. https://doi.org/10.1146/annurev.so.18.080192.001233
13. Correia T (2017) Revisiting medicalization: a critique of the assumptions of what counts as medical knowledge. Front Sociol 2. https://doi.org/10.3389/fsoc.2017.00014
14. Brownlee S, Chalkidou K, Doust J, Elshaug AG, Glasziou P, Heath I et al (2017) Evidence for overuse of medical services around the world. Lancet 390(10090):156–168. https://doi.org/10.1016/s0140-6736(16)32585-5
15. Busfield J (2017) The concept of medicalisation reassessed. Sociol Health Illn 39(5):759–774. https://doi.org/10.1111/1467-9566.12538
16. Ballard K, Elston MA (2005) Medicalisation: a multi-dimensional concept. Soc Theory Health 3(3):228–241. https://doi.org/10.1057/palgrave.sth.8700053
17. Martins C, Godycki-Cwirko M, Heleno B, Brodersen J (2018) Quaternary prevention: reviewing the concept: quaternary prevention aims to protect patients from medical harm. Eur J Gen Pract 24(1):106–111. https://doi.org/10.1080/13814788.2017.1422177
18. Bentzen N (2003) Wonca dictionary of general/family practice. Manedsskrift for Praktisk Laegergerning, Copenhagen
19. United Nation. Sustainable developmental goals. https://sdgs.un.org/goals
20. UN DESA (2022) The sustainable development goals report 2022 - July 2022. New York, USA: UN DESA. © UN DESA. https://unstats.un.org/sdgs/report/2022/
21. He J, Ortiz J (2021) Sustainable business modeling: the need for innovative design thinking. J Clean Prod 298(126751):126751. https://doi.org/10.1016/j.jclepro.2021.126751
22. Brennan A, Norva YSL (2002) Environmental ethics. In: Zalta EN (ed) The Stanford encyclopedia of philosophy. Stanford University, Stanford. https://plato.stanford.edu/archives/win2021/entries/ethics-environmental/
23. Soini K, Birkeland I (2014) Exploring the scientific discourse on cultural sustainability. Geoforum 51:213–223. https://doi.org/10.1016/j.geoforum.2013.12.001
24. Andrews D (2015) The circular economy, design thinking and education for sustainability. Local Econ 30(3):305–315. https://doi.org/10.1177/0269094215578226
25. Woods K (2010) Human rights and environmental sustainability. Edward Elgar Publishing, Cheltenham
26. Birkeland J (2012) Design blindness in sustainable development: from closed to open systems design thinking. J Urban Des 17(2):163–187. https://doi.org/10.1080/13574809.2012.666209
27. Hoolohan C, Brownie AL (2020) Design thinking for practice-based intervention: co-producing the charge points toolkit to unlock (un)sustainable practices. Des Stud 67:102–132
28. Shapira H, Ketchie A, Nehe M (2017) The integration of design thinking and strategic sustainable development. J Clean Prod 140:277–287. https://doi.org/10.1016/j.jclepro.2015.10.092
29. Pichler P-P, Jaccard IS, Weisz U, Weisz H (2019) International comparison of health care carbon footprints. Environ Res Lett 14(6):064004. https://doi.org/10.1088/1748-9326/ab19e1
30. Beauchamp TL, Childress JF (1992) Principles biomedical ethics. Oxford University Press, Cary, NC

31. The European code of conduct for research integrity (2019) Allea.org. ALLEA [cited 2022 Nov 9]. https://allea.org/code-of-conduct/
32. Nathan G (2015) Innovation process and ethics in technology: an approach to ethical (responsible) innovation governance. J Chain Netw Sci 15(2):119–134. https://doi.org/10.3920/jcns2014.x018
33. Blok V, Lemmens P (2015) The emerging concept of responsible innovation. Three reasons why it is questionable and calls for a radical transformation of the concept of innovation. In: Responsible innovation 2. Springer International Publishing, Cham, pp 19–35
34. The Lund Declaration (2009). https://www.vr.se/download/18.6969eb1a16a5b ec8b59338/1556886570218/Lund%20Declaration%202009.pdf
35. Pacifico Silva H, Lehoux P, Miller FA, Denis J-L (2018) Introducing responsible innovation in health: a policy-oriented framework. Health Res Policy Syst 16(1):90. https://doi.org/10.1186/s12961-018-0362-5
36. Owen R, Macnaghten P, Stilgoe J (2012) Responsible research and innovation: from science in society to science for society, with society. Sci Public Policy 39(6):751–760. https://doi.org/10.1093/scipol/scs093
37. Schomberg V (2013) A vision of responsible research and innovation. In: Owen R, Bessant J, Heintz M (eds) Responsible innovation. Wiley, London, pp 51–74

Design Thinking Toolkit for Healthcare Innovation

3

Beate Rygg Johnsen

3.1 Introduction

Too many ideas do not reach the market or users, even if the idea is good. This is often due to a suboptimal match between the product and the needs of the user, rather than the solution or technology itself being poor. It is difficult to foresee all preferences and conditions that are needed for an invention to come into use, and it is quite common that products end up having some unforeseen detail that may hinder its intended use.

We also tend to empathise more with similar individuals and not so much with groups of people with other needs than ourselves. It is difficult to stay objective when investigating someone else's situation without applying subjective assumptions. This typically applies to cases and situations that are far from our own everyday life.

In this chapter we suggest a toolbox of techniques that can help us stay objective through the design phase of a new product or service, that may prevent bias and does not require prior knowledge.

3.1.1 Simple Tools to Get You Started

Design thinking is a process that allows you to design your product or solution through the eyes of the user, securing a perfect fit between the solution and the end-user problem. The process is simply explained in Fig. 3.1. The first two steps, *empathy* and *define*, represent the problem finding phase. Steps three, four and five (*ideate*, *prototype* and *test*) represent the problem solving phase.

B. R. Johnsen (✉)
UiO Growth House, University of Oslo, Oslo, Norway
e-mail: beaterj@uio.no

A. Pakarinen et al. (eds.), *Design Thinking in Healthcare*,
https://doi.org/10.1007/978-3-031-24510-7_3

25

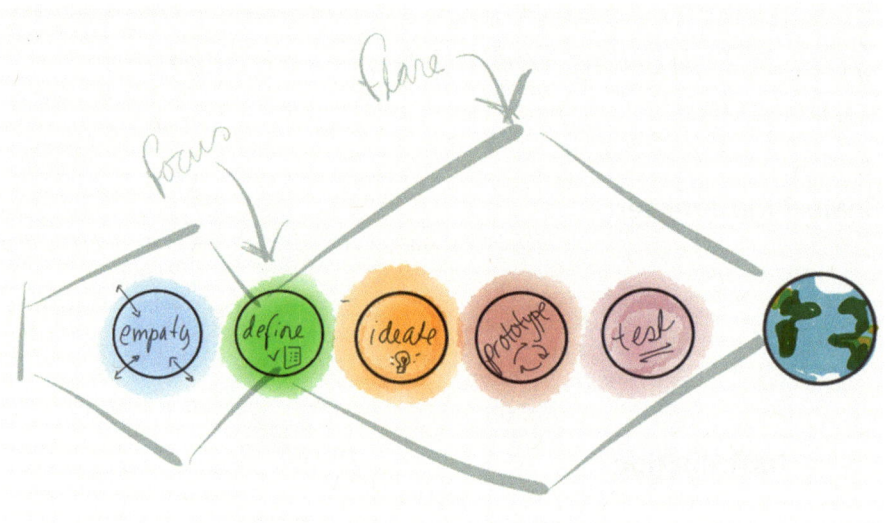

Fig. 3.1 The design thinking process—freely drawn from Stanford University and other graphics

The tools suggested in this chapter are only a few of many available ways to apply design thinking to an innovation process, but applying this selection of tools can help you stay open to the end-users' needs and create solutions that will solve a problem and hence be used. The chapter is organized in two main parts:

Part I: Problem Finding
- Observation, interviews and *job to be done*
- 5 whys
- Empathy map
- Point of view

Part II: Problem Solving
- How might we…
- Brainstorming
- Subtraction
- Prototype and test

3.2   Part I: Problem Finding

3.2.1   Observation, Interviews and the Job to Be Done

An important part of understanding a problem or need is observing and interviewing the users whose needs you seek to discover. Get yourself out there. Seek out the places where the needs manifest themselves.

A good source of understanding customer need is Clayton M. Christensen's description of the *job to be done* in his book *Competing Against Luck* (2016) [1]. In his book, Christensen describes the problem as *the job to be done* and the solution as something you *hire* to get the job done. In his book he describes that when McDonalds was looking to increase the sales of milkshakes, they turned immediately to introducing new flavours, new sizes, and so on but with little success. By investigating the people stopping by to buy milkshakes (their behaviour), they registered that milkshakes are particularly popular in the morning. They found that additional size and flavours did not increase sales, but that the morning milkshakes fill a specific purpose. Customers that stop before 9 a.m. are alone; they buy only milkshake and drive off. So, the question was: *what job are customers "hiring" the milkshake to do*? The customers could not answer directly, but through observation and interviews, it was revealed that they stopped to buy milkshake because they had a long commute to work and would otherwise be hungry by 10. When asked what could have been "hired" instead of a milkshake, they would suggest beagles, a banana, a Snickers bar, but these hires would leave crumbs, not be filling enough, be too sweet, and so on. Milkshake, on the other hand, would fit the bill perfectly. It was rich, was easy to handle, fit cup-holder, took time to drink and "keeps me full until lunch".

All shared a common "job to be done" in the morning. Afternoon buys have a different "job to be done", such as connecting with your children. It also has different, comparable and alternative "hires" such as going to the park or to a movie.

Observation is the first step to understanding people's true needs as people may find it difficult to express where the problem lies. To place yourself in the situation is key, and to try to replicate what the end-user is experiencing. The second step is *interviewing* people in these situations, and the following section will give some guidance in how to do this.

This part is especially important, because surprising as it is, people do not always know what their true needs are. If asked to describe a need, they jump straight to a solution they think might solve their problem. Influenced by others, and looking for solutions amongst already existing products, they struggle to see the best possible solution to a problem.

This is where you come in to guide and explore, and to do so, it is critical to *get close to people*. Understand their ways and their passions before you submerge yourself in discovering their struggles. They are the experts of their own problems, and you are the one trying to learn what it is all about. Normally you can only look to children close to you to understand the importance of this engagement. They often struggle with issues that we as adults cannot see but try to solve in our adult way. One simple example is trying to teach my 3-year-old the joys of downhill skiing. I tried to teach him how to do turns, but he seemed annoyed. When I sat down to engage with him, I realised that holding him back from going fast down the slope only delayed his big thrill, which was riding the ski tow to the top of the hill.

Observation and engagement is particularly important where children are concerned as they are often less skilled in articulating their needs or fears. One example described in Tom and David Kelley's book *Creative Confidence* [2], tells the story of how lead designer of GE Healthcare's new MRI machine, Doug Dietz, came to observe the MRI in use and discovered a young girl terrified of his new machine [3]. After the MRI had been taken into use, Doug learned that most kids were scared and as much as 80% of them needed to be sedated to keep still during the procedure. Horrified by this statistics, Doug decided to fix this problem and sought training in design thinking. The human-centred method gave him the skills to engage with children and their caretakers to understand how kids experience, and interact with, technology. Through his "anthropological fieldwork" and a creative problem solving process (methodology described later in this chapter), Doug transformed the MRI suite into an "adventure story". He painted MRI machines as pirate ships, space capsules and submarines and prepared scripts for the operators, making the kids captains of their vessels. Doug's empathy-based innovation helped reduce the sedation of paediatric patients down to a handful and changed kids' experience from utter horror to an adventure (Fig. 3.2).

Your role, in addition to observing behaviour, is to ask questions that will unveil what hinders them in their work or daily life. The most important part of asking questions is to keep an open mind, listen to and build on the answers you receive, rather than bringing a list of pre-prepared questions. From a simple topic, let the user take you into his or her world and try to understand what their story is and how the problem makes them feel. Below is a list of some simple tips when asking questions:

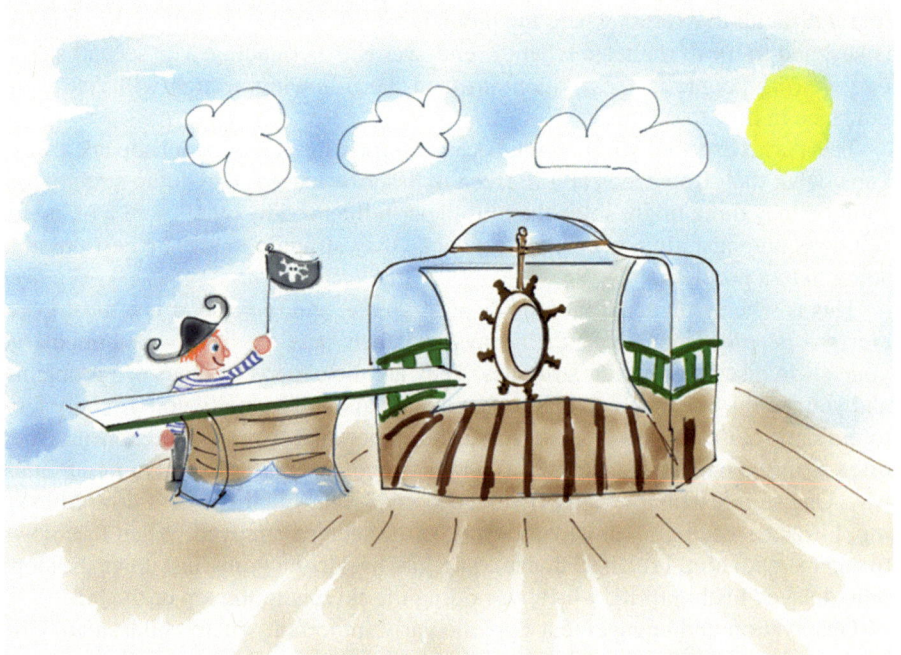

Fig. 3.2 GE Healthcare's new, improved MRI "adventure"

- Begin very basic and ask short open questions ("can you help me out …").
- Be specific about situation that comes up:
  - What is the problem?
  - When did you last have this problem?
  - What were you feeling?
  - What happened?
- Ask why for statements like "I think" or "I believe".
- Give ample time to reflect and answer—silence is OK.
- Bring with you someone who can make notes and capture the interview.

Although the morning milkshake represents an incremental improvement to a marketed product, what the story tells us is the importance of understanding your customer or user's true need. This is the case whether you have a specific idea in mind or whether you see an unfulfilled need in the market. In the case of a product idea, the first you must do is to put your invention aside and visit the segment where you think your idea will provide value. When you investigate the need/problems, also look at what users currently do to minimise the problem.

In the case of a market need or unsolved problem, the first phase is empathising with the user. In the healthcare segment, a problem or need can be anything from a marketed solution that is too comprehensive and thus not being used, a solution that is too expensive, too complicated or not anatomically compatible with all users or maybe an instrument that is scary to kids.

3.2.2 5 Whys

When meeting with new environments, it is sometimes difficult to start asking open questions without bias toward answers that you expect will come. In these instances, it can be good to have a proven questioning technique to lean on. One such technique is the 5 whys technique. It was originally developed by Toyota industries in the 1930s as a method to find the root cause of a manufacturing problem. Toyota still uses this method and today it is widely used in lean manufacturing, e.g. to perform root cause analysis or eliminate wasteful manufacturing processes.

The technique is very simple. You simply ask "why" when someone tells you about a situation from his or her experience. After five whys you will have come to the origin of the problem. Example:

An elderly malnourished person living at home: "I cannot seem to maintain my weight"—WHY—"I cannot find food that I like"—WHY—"I only buy ready-made food that doesn't taste so good"—WHY—"I prefer vegetables, but the good food is too hard to prepare"—WHY—"I cannot use sharp knives and peelers to prepare the veggies"—WHY—"my hands are too weak to grip the tools and cut the hard veggies". Aha!

As consumers cannot always articulate what they want, this is where the 5 WHYs and other interviewing techniques come in handy. In addition to asking questions unveiling whether a user will buy a product or service (what Clayton M. Christensen would call the *big hire*), one should also keep in mind whether the product will be used after the purchase is done. This, referred to as the "little hire", and is not often investigated, even in design thinking. To ensure that you have captured the problem correctly so that a potential product or service will fill a purpose also after it has been "hired", one can test this by completing the following sentence by filling in the (*blanks*):

WHEN: __(*a situation occurs*)__ I WANT TO:__ (*motivation*)___ SO I CAN:_ (*expected outcome*)___.

E.g. when I am hungry I want to be able to eat vegetables so I can maintain my weight.

3.2.3 Empathy Map

After you and your team have gathered observations and answers to interviews, it is time to structure the data and findings. The purpose being that with the task of structuring and interpretation you will arrive at some *insights* about the problem and situation at hand.

Start by asking the team to put all their answers and observations on post-it notes (Fig. 3.3). You may discuss along the way to reflect and remember all elements. Then group the notes from all team members into similar answers and observations. Arrange a large piece of blank paper or wall into four squares and put your observations and answers/statements on the left side.

On the right side of the empathy map, you discuss the following in the team: behind the statements and observations; what do you think are the users' true thoughts and feelings. Do your own interpretation of what they say and do. What do

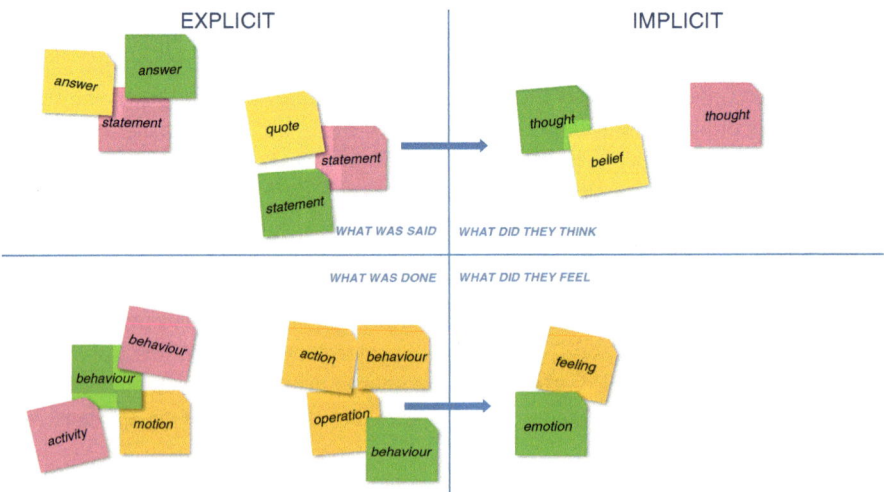

Fig. 3.3 Empathy map: freely drawn from Stanford University model

you think are their beliefs and true thoughts ("I wonder if this means …")? Are there any surprises or new thoughts that spring from working with transitioning pure observation into inferences—what are these new *insights*?

Through your interpretations of what you hear and the *insights* you have discovered, you may reveal issues that you did not think of starting out. Moreover, keep in mind that it is OK to speculate and make assumptions, as the validity of these insights will be tested later on in the process. These possible insights are now the source of your *point of view* (POV) sentence.

3.2.4 Point of View

To form a *Point of View* (POV) is to frame a challenge that will be the starting point for entering the *solution* phase of the design process. The POV is an actionable problem statement that is the cumulation of all the work done in the empathising phase. It is a crystalised form of one version of the problem as you and your team see it. As defined by Professor James A. Landay at Stanford University, a POV statement is:

> A unique, concise reframing of the problem that is grounded in user needs & insights
> —Professor James A. Landay

But be aware, it is NOT a consensus of the behaviours of all people who are experiencing this problem in all its shapes and forms, but a focus on one selected meaningful challenge.

To frame the POV, ask yourself the following sentences:

- Who did you meet?
- What were you surprised to notice?
- What do you "wonder if it means"?
- What would be game-changing?

The first sentence captures a person or the synthesis of people that experience the problem in one way. In this situation, it can be useful to choose an extreme user with an "exaggerated" problem to emphasise the issue. Extreme in the sense demographic, psychographic or other. Demographic means someone's race, ethnicity, religious beliefs, age, occupation, income, social class and education level, whereas psychographics refers to consumers based on their activities, interests and opinions. Choose one angle to the problem and define what surprised you. Then add your interpretation of what you think this means—what was inferred, what needs you discovered. In the final sentence, frame the game-changing challenge in the way of an *informed* problem that is specific to your person. A good POV should inspire your team, capture the people you have met and provide focus and frame the next phase.

In the case of the elderly malnourished person, one POV could be:

- "the elderly want to eat fresh vegetables without having to use standard cutting utensils" or
- "the elderly want to eat normal, but are limited by their aging bodies"

It is important *not to limit* the problem by introducing solutions into the POV, e.g.:

- "the elderly need a new type of cutting utensils to be able to eat fresh vegetables".

Most importantly, no matter which approach of interviews or observation you use, the time-consuming task of putting yourself out there and talking to the users in the development phase is of the essence. A recent review of *usability challenges and medical devices in the home environment* revealed that only 12 out of the 3471 studies reviewed had direct involvement of end-users [4]. The lack of user involvement, they found, resulted in machines with complex feedback systems that also lacked intuitiveness in use. The home environment is less structured and consists of a broad user range. Omitting user involvement increases the likelihood of adverse events.

3.3   Part II: Problem Solving

Allegedly, Henry Ford is known to have said:

> If I had asked people what they wanted, they would have said faster horses
> —Henry Ford

Although this statement might be more an anecdote than a fact, it brilliantly points to the fact that we humans are limited by our automatic thoughts. We tend to seek solutions within our prior knowledge when faced with a problem.

Design thinking is all about managing a state of ambiguity. Finding and solving problems in a state of uncertainty also means managing discomfort. You are not looking for a pre-set answer, but finding the best possible solution amongst an ocean of potential, so far unknown solutions. You must go through the discomfort of not knowing the answer and be creative and explorative in this state in order to arrive at new discoveries.

Design is getting from problem finding to problem solving and to quote Justin Ferrell of Stanford d.school; "you must dare to *endure, engage* and *embrace* ambiguity to make your path to a unique discovery".

Problem solving, that is, finding a solution, may bring an additional dimension of discomfort. In creating an ideal situation for the creative process, you must strive to put together a team that is as diverse as possible. Try to create some points of collision in the way you assemble your team consisting of people with different scientific and cultural backgrounds that see the world in different ways and have different values and virtues. This because "hiring individuals who do not look, talk, or think like you can allow you to dodge the costly pitfalls of conformity, which discourages innovative thinking" [5].

The significance of the diverse team and managing ambiguity are key elements when moving into phase three, the ideation phase. This phase is all about coming up with as many ideas as possible, and so we must trust the founder of design thinking, David Kelley, and believe his statement:

Belief in your creative capacity lies at the heart of innovation
   —David Kelley

3.3.1   How Might We

The POV from the last section can be framed into "how might we …" statements (HMWs) to spark the ideation phase, that is, how might we accomplish the game changer. The how might we statements are not closed and definite, but open and inviting you to frame a sentence that addresses the POV. In the case of the elderly, malnourished person, a HMW statement could be "how might we create new tools so that this person could peel and cut her veggies" or "how might we supply her with fresh pre-cut vegetables" or "how might we make pre-cooked meals more tasty". The point is to explore the POV from all angles when creating HMW statements by brainstorming as many solutions as possible. Introducing alternatives to all parts of the problem such as, the who, what, when, where and so on.

3.3.2   Brainstorming

Brainstorming is one technique/tool that can be used to come up with HMW statements. The first rule of brainstorming ideas is quantity over quality. To find one or two surprisingly inventive ideas, one must generate a plethora of ideas. The wilder and more diverse the better.

This is where the diversity of the team is key and creating a safe environment for people to speak freely without judgement. It is forbidden in this part of the process, to disagree or contradict and idea, but it is encouraged to add to the ideas of others, for example, by adding a "yes, and …" to someone's statement. You'll need plenty of empty walls and post-it notes. Allow plenty of time to make HMW statements on post-it notes and take timeouts where you explain your ideas to the others allowing the idea to develop through building on each other's ideas.

Due to the diversity of the team, there should also be some rules for the brainstorming session. This is not to suffocate creativity, but to allow all ideas to surface:

- Take turns speaking so all voices are heard.
- One person at a time.
- To maintain energy and speed, keep your idea description at a headline level.

3.3.3   Subtraction

Sometimes, in brainstorming sessions, it might happen that ideas tend to evolve around the same topic and you may feel stuck. For example, all ideas may revolve around creating a new resource, and no ideas are creating analogies, question assumptions, explore opposites, changing status quo, and so on. One way to ignite a brainstorming session that is moving slow, is to introduce restrictions.

One such restriction is *subtraction*. In subtraction you use the POV as normal, but remove a vital part from the equation. This leaves you to *invent around* a subject that would normally be your focus. To illustrate, if we return to Henry Ford and his speedy horses, the subtraction made was that people still needed to get from A to B more quickly, but now without the horse. Henry Ford saw that the limitation was the horse itself, so he started to brainstorming (we might imagine) how to invent around using the horse all together, and ended up with a radically innovative solution. Similarly, in 2009 in San Francisco, Uber revolutionised busy city transportation by subtracting taxis from the equation. In the case of the malnourished person, one could easily get stuck inventing only new ergonomically correct tools for peeling vegetables. To use subtraction, one could take the utensil out of the equation. This would spark new ways of thinking and new solutions.

This is a powerful innovation tool. It also allows you to remove something from the equation that you would prefer to get rid of. *If* successful, this is a way to create disruptive ideas because it so radically changes the premises of the creation process.

Other tools to spur the brainstorming can be to introduce less dramatic restrictions to overcome the paralysis of having too many choices. These restrictions can be anything related or unrelated to the task, e.g. "the design must cost less than $100" or "the idea must fit into a pocket" or "be reusable". The purpose is to help your brain think in new directions or to introduce a clear preference.

When you have emptied the creative process, take one step back and arrange the ideas into themes. Agree in your team on logical ways to group the HMW statements. Then agree on how to select the ideas you want to move to the phase four: prototyping. You may choose to select themes or single ideas. Ways to select ideas should be *democratic*. Each person gets a defined number of votes and places a sticker-dot on their favourites. It is also possible to have different colour dots for far-fetched ideas and low hanging fruit if you would like to select ideas with different risk-profiles for testing.

3.3.4   Prototype and Test

Prototyping is an iterative process where you test your ideas with the users. The purpose is to collect data on all three aspects of an innovation (Fig. 3.4):

- Technical feasibility: can we make it?
- Market desirable: does someone need it and want it?
- Business viability: can we make money on it?

Fig. 3.4 Free drawing from Stanford University model

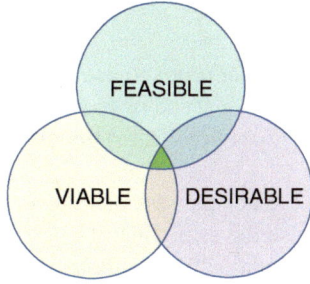

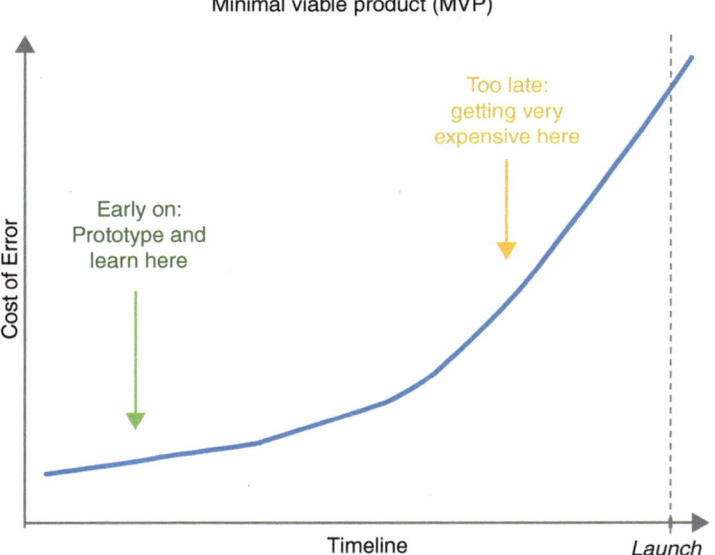

Fig. 3.5 Free drawing inspired by Stanford University

The effort you put into the prototype will grow linearly with the conviction you get from the response you collect, that this is a good idea (middle triangle in the chart). The viability aspect is saved for last as it is more elaborate to document.

Start simple. If you put too much effort in your prototype, you tend to cherish and build on it, which may create bias. Also, the time it takes to make a "perfect" prototype, prevents you from making changes fast and produces multiple iterations and also controlling cost (Fig. 3.5). Rather build the cheapest and simplest possible mock-up of what your solution will look like when you start testing. Be creative. Examples of prototypes include simple drawings or post-its, descriptive leaflets, cardboard 3D models or any material that can be built into something recognisable and representative.

Next, create the time and space for your experiments to test the various prototypes.

Plan:

- What props to use?
- What scene or space will your experiment take place in?
- Assign roles for people to play during the test/roleplays.

Keep the sessions short and defined and collect as many experiments as possible. Use the same line of questioning from *the problem finding* section above. One role should be to take thorough notes and pictures when possible and allowed.

When you have tested the prototype, go back and make necessary alterations based on the feedback, then test again until you feel that you have a prototype worth exploring further that can be continued in the product design phase.

3.4   Conclusion

Designing products and solutions to meet the users' true needs is all about stepping into the unknown. A prerequisite for managing such a "risky" situation is to embrace the uncomfortableness of not knowing where you are going and be confident that you and your team's creative thinking will get you there. It is as much a mindset as a defined process. And remember, you are not a failure if you fail to excel the first time around. You are just wiser and better skilled to tackle your next round of innovation by design thinking.

Acknowledgments   A big thanks to Norunn Torheim and Nicolay Bérard-Andersen for reviewing and commenting on the text, and for great collaboration in our task to introduce design-driven innovation to academia.

References

1. Christensen CM et al (2016) Competing against luck—the story of innovation and customer choice. Harper Business, New York
2. Kelley T, Kelley D (2013) Creative confidence—unleashing the creative potential within us all. Crown, New York
3. Dietz D (2012) Transforming healthcare for children and their families. TEDx San Jose, CA. https://youtu.be/jajduxPD6H4. Accessed 30 Sep 2022
4. Tase A et al (2022) Usability challenges in the use of medical devices in the home environment: a systematic review of literature. Appl Ergon 103:103769
5. Rock D, Grant H (2016) Why diverse teams are smarter. Harv Bus Rev, November 4

Design Thinking in Healthcare Education

4

Isabella Hajduk, Annika Nordberg, and Eeva Rainio

4.1   A Brief History of Design Thinking in Education

The concept of Design Thinking originated in the 1960's to describe the collective problem-solving process that the professional (industrial) designers use when developing new products for consumers. Since then, it has also been integrated into higher education. Design Thinking is a widely used approach especially in business, marketing, and entrepreneurship education, but also in engineering, architecture, and other design areas. It has also recently, during the past 5 years (also based on authors' own observations), started to become an increasingly important pedagogical tool in the education of health professionals [1–3].

We have collected representative examples of how Design Thinking is used or taught in health education around the world, as shown in Table 4.1 at the end of the chapter. The table does not aim to be a complete listing, but rather gives inspiration for further reading. For more examples, we also recommend the following recent review articles to readers. Sandars and Goh offer recommendations, how to efficiently use Design Thinking in medical education. They have concluded that Design Thinking usually has two main uses: it has been used directly to design a new product, or the principles of Design Thinking have been taught to students with the help

I. Hajduk
The Centre for Innovative Medical Research, Sydney, NSW, Australia
e-mail: isabella.hajduk@cimrglobal.com

A. Nordberg
Department of Nursing Science, University of Turku, Turku, Finland

E. Rainio (✉)
Faculty of Medicine, University of Turku, Turku, Finland
e-mail: eeva.rainio@utu.fi

© The Author(s), under exclusive license to Springer Nature
Switzerland AG 2023
A. Pakarinen et al. (eds.), *Design Thinking in Healthcare*,
https://doi.org/10.1007/978-3-031-24510-7_4

Table 4.1 Examples of how Design Thinking is used in health education

How was Design Thinking used?	References
Curriculum and course development	
Design Thinking was used in curriculum development: Since 2015 at Harvard Medical School the students have participated in curriculum work. They are, after all, the end users of the "product", which is the course curriculum	Anderson, J., Calahan, C.F. & Gooding, H. (2017): Applying design thinking to curriculum reform. *Academic Medicine* 92(4), 427
Design Thinking process was used to create a course Design Thinking for Public Good for public health students at the University of North Carolina at Chapel Hill	Skywark, E. R., Chen, E., & Jagannathan, V. (2021). Using the design thinking process to co-create a new, interdisciplinary design thinking course to train 21st century graduate students. *Frontiers in Public Health, 9*
A full-day Design Thinking retreat to rethink the needs for continuing professional education with emergency medicine stakeholders	Chorley, A., Azzam, K., & Chan, T. M. (2020). Redesigning continuing professional development: Harnessing design thinking to go from needs assessment to mandate. *Perspectives on Medical Education, 1–6*
Design Thinking process was used in a 2-day workshop for health profession educators to develop recommendations how to evaluate the interprofessional health education	Cahn, P. S., Bzowyckyj, A., Collins, L., Dow, A., Goodell, K., Johnson, A. F., ... & Zierler, B. K. (2016). A design thinking approach to evaluating interprofessional education. *Journal of Interprofessional Care*, 30(3), 378–380
Design Thinking was used to solve an educational problem: how to overcome challenges with rural placements of students in various health professions	Wolcott, M. D., McLaughlin, J. E., Hubbard, D. K., Williams, C. R., & Kiser, S. N. (2021). Using design thinking to explore rural experiential education barriers and opportunities. *Journal of Medical Education and Curricular Development*, 8, 2382120521992333
Clinical Experience program was improved at Sidney Kimmel Medical College in a 3-h Design Thinking sprint with the program stakeholders. As a result, changes were introduced, and significant improvement of student satisfaction achieved	Fish, A. M., Fields, J. M., Ziring, D., McCoy, G., Ostroff, P., & Hayden, G. (2022). Curriculum development by design thinking: Analyzing a program for social determinants of health screening by pre-clerkship medical students. *Journal of Medical Education and Curricular Development*, 9, 23821205221080701
A novel online educational resource, The Path to Patient-Centred Care was developed with the support of a Design Jam event	MacKinnon, K. R., Ross, L. E., Rojas Gualdron, D., & Ng, S. L. (2020). Teaching health professionals how to tailor gender-affirming medicine protocols: a design thinking project. *Perspectives on Medical Education*, 9(5), 324–328

Table 4.1 (continued)

How was Design Thinking used?	References
Nursing education/interprofessional education in nursing	
Transdisciplinary course to engineering, nursing, and pre-professional health students was organized to introduce them to novel technologies and innovate solutions for community health problems. The course utilized MakerSpace open learning environment for prototyping. Special emphasis was on increasing understanding about ethical implications related to novel technologies	Lewis, E. J., Ludwig, P. M., Nagel, J., & Ames, A. (2019). Student ethical reasoning confidence pre/post an innovative makerspace course: A survey of ethical reasoning. *Nurse Education Today*, 75, 75–79
Presents a pilot of an innovation and Design Thinking workshop for nursing and sustainable peacebuilding students with the help of University Entrepreneurship Center at the Midwestern University's College of Nursing. The aim was to expose students to Design Thinking and teach them to use creativity and innovation	Holt, J. M., Talsma, A., Woehrle, L. M., Klingbeil, C., & Avdeev, I. Fostering innovation and design thinking in graduate programs. *Nurse Educator*, 10–1097
The article provides insights how the nursing faculty at the University of Alabama at Birmingham has used Design Thinking in introducing nursing research to undergraduate students. They discuss the Design Thinking benefits reflected in student experiences, including understanding the empathy in healthcare and future potential of understanding the Design Thinking process	Wingo, N., Jones, C. R., Pittman, B. R., Purter, T., Russell, M., Brown, J., & Ladores, S. (2020). Applying design thinking in health care: Reflections of nursing honors program students. *Creative Nursing*, 26(3), 169–174
Gives an example of interdisciplinary healthcare design jam event on the theme of innovative thinking to support LGBTQI2S Health and Wellness. In addition, the authors continued the development of an online education tool kit by partnering with nurse researchers who develop simulation games for nurses	Ziegler, E., Carroll, B., & Shortall, C. (2020). Design Thinking in nursing education to improve care for lesbian, gay, bisexual, transgender, queer, intersex and two-spirit people. *Creative Nursing*, 26(2), 118–124
Nursing students in South Korea were taught patient-centered care (PCC) with the help of 5-step Design Thinking process, 2 h each. After the course they self-evaluated their views on supporting patient individuality and on maintaining patient individuality while providing care. Results showed that student understanding about PCC increased during the program	Park, M., Giap, T. T. T., Jang, I., Jeong, M., & Kim, J. (2022, January). Listening to patients' voices: Applying the design-thinking method for teaching person-centered care to nursing students. In *Nursing Forum* (Vol. 57, no. 1, pp. 9–17)

(continued)

Table 4.1 (continued)

How was Design Thinking used?	References
Interprofessional education in other health disciplines	
Paper describes a use of Design Thinking process in an abridged hackathon workshop to promote interprofessional and inter-clinic collaboration on student-run clinics, as well as encourage workshop participants to design clinic practice improvements	Chen, K., Kruger, J., McCarther, N., & Meah, Y. (2020). Interprofessional, learner-driven collaboration for innovative solutions to healthcare delivery in student-run clinics. *Journal of Interprofessional Care*, 34(1), 137–139
Design Thinking principles were utilized in designing a shift handoff software as an interprofessional collaborative effort of medical informatics program and school of architecture and design	Lesselroth, B., Park, H., Duncan, H. M. A., Thompson, G., & Yarnall, R. (2021). Designing shift handoff software: Clinical learners and design students collaborate using the "design thinking" process. *Studies in Health Technology and Informatics*, 281, 974–978
This paper gives an example of Design Thinking Community Medicine workshop to teach about health-related social needs and to practice designing person-centered solutions for medical and physician assistant students	Lesselroth, B., Park, H., Monkman, H., Ijams, S., Yarnall, R., Kollaja, L., & Dennis, S. (2021). Student academy: A pilot design thinking workshop to teach community medicine. In context sensitive health informatics: The role of informatics in global pandemics (pp. 79–83). IOS Press.
Stanford University d.school offered Medical Device Design workshops to multidisciplinary team of undergraduate and graduate students: engineering, design, medicine, business, law, humanities, education, and earth sciences. They compared the experiential and observational learning during the first two phases of Design Thinking: understanding and defining the problems	Sherman, J., Lee, H. C., Weiss, M. E., & Kristensen-Cabrera, A. (2018). Medical device design education: identifying problems through observation and hands-on training. *Design and technology education: An International Journal*, 23(2), 154
Medical education	
3-day Innovation and Design Thinking course was piloted as a mandatory course in Singapore, aiming to give the medical students an overview of healthcare innovation, let them create their own solutions in design sprint, and practice pitching	Chen, P. P. Y., & Chou, A. C. C. (2021). Teaching health care innovation to medical students. *The Clinical Teacher*, 18(3), 285–289
University of Virginia offers Design Thinking course for first-year medical students. During this course, which lasts 1 year, the students will develop new services and solutions for patient work. This module had a clearly positive impact on their learning throughout the rest of their studies	Trowbridge, M., Chen, D. & Gregor, A. 2018: Teaching design thinking to medical students. *Medical Education* 52, 1199–1200

Table 4.1 (continued)

How was Design Thinking used?	References
In 2017 AMEE, an event called #ElsevierHacks utilizing Design Thinking methodology was carried out with students. It lasted 48 h, and together with software developers and designers the students generated new tools, such as mobile phone apps, to help with challenges in medical education. The participating teams also received support from marketing and technology specialists, as well as from medical educators Authors stated that Design Thinking gives excellent lifelong learning skills, which assist with teamwork and tolerating uncertainty, two very basic characteristics common to all healthcare professions	Badwan, B., Bothara, R., Latijnhouwers, M., Smithies, A. & Sandars, J. 2018: The importance of design thinking in medical education. *Medical Teacher* 40(4), 425–426
Design Thinking methodology has also turned out to be useful in trainings, where students solve complex ethical issues. This paper describes a Design Thinking workshop to propose better alternatives for liver transplant allocation system in US	Marcus, D., Simone, A., & Block, L. (2020). Design thinking in medical ethics education. *Journal of Medical Ethics*, 46(4), 282–284
Online transition examples from COVID-19 pandemic	
Description of teaching methods and learning outcomes from a novel course for American biomedical engineering and natural sciences students who participated on study-abroad activities in both US and Portugal. Aim was to teach how culture impacts on healthcare delivery and use of technologies The course went through a transition from study-abroad to study-online during COVID-19, and changes were reported in this article	Ferreira, M. F., Savoy, J. N., & Markey, M. K. (2020). Teaching cross-cultural design thinking for healthcare. *The Breast*, 50, 1–10 Lewis, M. M., & Markey, M. K. (2021). From study-abroad to study-at-home: teaching cross-cultural design thinking during COVID-19. *Biomedical Engineering Education*, 1(1), 121–125
University of Pennsylvania School of Nursing transitioned their hands-on community service course Innovations in Health: Foundations of Design Thinking, to online course and report the course changes and outcomes	Karwat, A., Richmond, T. S., & Leary, M. (2021). Transition of a collaborative in-person health care innovation course to online learning. *Journal of Nursing Education*, 60(5), 298–300

of a project where the participants develop a new product [4]. The nature of a new product can vary from curriculum reforms to medical applications. In their commentary, Madson summarizes the operationalization of current understandings of Design Thinking in medical education. They introduce different initiatives to incorporate Design Thinking into the curriculum [5]. Madson divides them into education programs, courses, workshops, and hackathons, from more extensive modules to short training events. Inspired by these reviews, the examples in the table are divided according to the use of Design Thinking in curriculum/content development or in educational courses/trainings. In addition, the references are grouped based on the field of education.

4.2   About the Chapter's Authors

Isabella, Eeva, and Annika all come from science/medical backgrounds, where Isabella is a molecular microbiologist, Eeva is a geneticist, and Annika is a nursing scientist. Throughout their academic careers, they each have had the opportunity to contribute to the teaching and learning side of tertiary education.

During her PhD candidature at the University of Technology Sydney (UTS) in Australia, Isabella was given an opportunity to participate in an international training program in the area of biomedical innovation and entrepreneurship (BIE), run by Professor Michael Wallach. The 2-week intense program takes a Design Thinking approach, where students are tasked with defining a health or medical problem and ideating and pitching an innovative and novel solution. Students are supported with relevant education and expert-mentoring throughout the program to help shape their ideas into feasible solutions. The BIE course was later adapted into a Master's core subject, called Innovation, Entrepreneurship, and Commercialization (IEC). Isabella joined Professor Wallach in teaching IEC in 2016, and since took an active role in further elevating the IEC subject into a fun, educational subject marrying biomedical sciences and Design Thinking.

Eeva was first introduced to the Design Thinking approach on a career course and fell in love with the approach. After visiting Stanford d.school in 2019, she was convinced that the Faculty of Medicine at the University of Turku needs to learn more about Design Thinking. Eeva's final project during her pedagogics studies in 2020 was a short Design Thinking course for medical students to assist them with their personal study plans. She was also the brains behind a new Design Thinking course concept called GREAT. She wrote a successful grant to Nordic Council of Ministers, which helped the Faculty of Medicine to organize its first multidisciplinary health and nursing-focused Design Thinking course, Design Future Health, or GREAT.

Annika is a public health nurse, whose passion has always been in the improvement of patients and end users experience. She has a shiny new Master's degree diploma in Health Sciences, graduated from the University of Turku. Annika has had experiences in design thinking courses on both sides: she took part in the international version of the BIE course in 2020 as a student and has also worked as a project coordinator and teacher in the above-mentioned GREAT, as well as in a very similar course called D.pop, which is intended for the healthcare professionals.

This chapter is posed to be a guide and insight from teachers for teachers, for the integration of Design Thinking into STEM (Science, Technology, Engineering, Mathematics) education with some tools and exercises to be used by teachers. It will be described predominantly in context of the IEC course at UTS and the BIE course, and the lessons learned by Isabella, with additional insight from Eeva and Annika and their experiences in the GREAT Course. This chapter is anecdotal in nature; however, since its inception in 2012, there have been many iterations and improvements to the IEC course, with much feedback from the students and many lessons learned, which the authors have shared here.

4.3   About Our Courses

The IEC course is run over 12 weeks in a connected progressive manner and delivered in three progressive themes: team building, science, and business. The BIE course is much like the IEC course; however, it is delivered in a 2-week intensive mode. The students are posed with a health or medical problem, which over the course of the subject, they need to break down and develop for it a hypothetical but feasible solution. The problems put forward are ones from academics at the university in their area of research. These academics participate several times throughout the subject to provide mentorship and feedback, ensuring that the ideas being developed are scientifically feasible and uphold established dogmas of the topic. This mentorship is one of the key factors for successful learning and engagement for the students, which will be discussed more later.

Design Future Health or GREAT was a combination of a 4-week course held online and a week-long intensive course, intended for both MSc and PhD students representing multiple fields including nursing science, medicine, biomedicine, pharmacy, information science, health technology, and economics. The student groups received real-life challenges collected from healthcare services, and over the courses they solved them following the Design Thinking process. The course aimed to equip the participants with a new way of creative thinking about complex healthcare problems and also increase their entrepreneurial mindset.

4.3.1   How Best to Deliver a Design Thinking Course?

A key lesson from teaching these courses is that nothing is certain, and we need to take on uncertainty and learn to pivot. The COVID-19 pandemic was undoubtedly an event of uncertainty and we had to quickly adapt and pivot our teaching approaches to different learning modes: in-person learning, solely online, or a hybrid approach. The hybrid approach can be interpreted in two ways: a mixed delivery approach where lectures are delivered online and workshops or other activities are delivered in-person; or where the classes are delivered in-person; however, the students can join either in-person or online. Table 4.2 provides an overview of the strengths and weaknesses that we have perceived firsthand from running our courses in different modes. Regarding hybrid, the strengths and weaknesses posed are in reference to the latter interpretation of hybrid delivery defined above.

While online has its clear advantages, social interaction is one of the most important factors for learning (especially Design Thinking) that is rooted in human experience. Isabella has run both programs, the BIE course and the IEC subject in each of the three modes. In her experience, Isabella believes in-person learning is the most effective mode of learning—both for the students and for the teachers. The students can establish a deeper connection with each other, while the teachers can directly sense when groups or students need help.

Running the programs online decreases the personal responsibility for engagement in the work. For example, in the BIE course, students will partake often from

Table 4.2 An overview of the strengths and weaknesses of different learning modes

	Face-to-face (classroom)	Online course	Hybrid
Strengths	• Allows for more extensive collaboration • Conducive to teamwork • Social interaction and network • Personalities can be expressed more freely • Allows for innovative group dynamics • Easy communication • Conducive to pre- and post-class discussion • Allows for coffee breaks, leading to further social interactions • More flexible content delivery • Teacher can help to motivate & encourage	• Flexible time frame (schedule) • Allows for attendance worldwide • Cost-effective for the organisers • Affordable for the attendees • Comfortable and convenient • Time efficient as there is no need to travel or set up classrooms • Easy access to digital learning materials	• Flexibility for all students, notably international students that are unable to reach the place of education for different reasons • Teachers do not need to repeat content for absentees because they are able to join the class online if they are sick • Opens opportunity to include international speakers for the educational material • Can be beneficial for the empathising stage of Design Thinking
Weaknesses	• Requires a dedicated location and space to which all parties need to travel. • Strict time schedule • Higher cost • Greater organisation efforts • For the block mode, there is a greater time commitment as it requires students to travel away from their place of work for a set time with little chance of completing some of their own work outside of the course hours	• Requires technology experience • Heightened chance of technical problems • Difficulty in having meaningful interaction with students • Difficulty in networking with others • Limited communal synergies • Different personalities may be perceived differently • Limited verbal/non-verbal communication	• Difficult to facilitate groups that have both in-person and online students. Online students are often left out of the conversations • Presentation of learning material requires the teacher to be connected with in-person and online students. Questions and interactions with online students are often left secondary • Classroom needs to be set up for hybrid (speakers, microphones, etc.) • Need to try and group students by their attendance mode and avoid mixing online with in person – leads to difficulty in communication and group discussion within the class

their place of work. Because of this, they often will take breaks away from the course to attend to other work. This adds a significant level of difficulty for the teacher to ascertain when the students require assistance or are just not present at their computers for the course. Running the courses face-to-face allows the students to focus on their team and the course work more actively.

Another factor to consider is the duration of the programs. We have each run our program over different durations:

1. BIE course: 2-week intensive, running full time (Monday to Friday, 9–4 pm; delivered either in-person or online only).
2. Great Course: hybrid mode—4 weeks online once a week for lessons to learn the fundamentals of Design Thinking, plus online group work with a real healthcare-related problem. After this introductory 4 weeks, 1 week in-person intensive mode where the application of Design Thinking method can be deepened with a new complex healthcare problem.
3. IEC subject: 3 h per week over 12 weeks. This is time spent with the teacher and does not include the hours that students spend together outside of class or completing assessments—this would average to be an additional 3 h per week. Has been delivered in all modes (in-person, online only, and hybrid).

Each of the three durations we have run has their advantages and disadvantages; however, it ultimately comes down to the requirements of the institutions and availability of the students.

4.4   A Student's Journey Through Design Thinking

Over the many years of running the three programs, we have observed an interesting journey or transition that the students go through over the duration of the course. That is, their experience within the classroom and within themselves parallels that of the journey through Design Thinking, going from problem to solution (Fig. 4.1). These three stages we have put forward as confusion, clarity, and completion: i) confusion: in who they are as an individual, how they can fit and contribute within

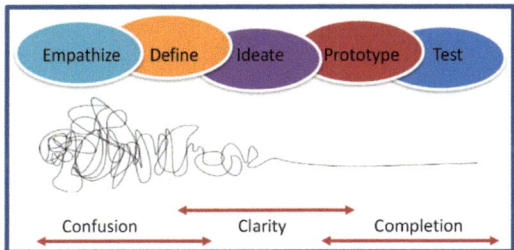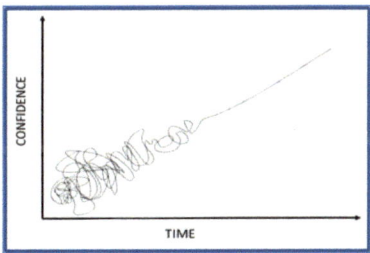

Fig. 4.1 Student's journey from confusion to completion and confidence during a typical Design Thinking course

a group setting, and their abilities in addressing complex and unfamiliar problems; ii) clarity: gaining confidence within themselves, in their creativity and contribution to the team, as well as their understanding of the problem and how to address it in a meaningful way; and iii) completion: the sense of achievement when they have worked together and to their strengths to put forward a well-developed, well-tested, and feasible solution.

One of the most reoccurring points of feedback we receive from students after completing our programs is that it is completely different to anything else they have done throughout their educational journey. They perfectly reiterate the stages mentioned above, highlighting how confused they are at the beginning, but then feel rewarded at the end. This is because the Design Thinking experience can be a difficult one to adapt to as it is a different way to learn. It is therefore ultimately our mission as the teacher to instill confidence in the students and push them out of their comfort zones to achieve something they have not done before. This is ultimately essential for their own personal and professional growth, leading them to:

- Take more risks
- Ask questions
- Think critically
- Think outside the box
- Encourage a desire for lifelong learning
- Expand their thinking in generating ideas and seeing them through
- Improve their communication skills

All these factors ultimately culminate to better healthcare professionals. Employers are increasingly seeking individuals with a range of soft skills that can be deployed within teams and entire organizations, including creativity, adaptability, communication, management, and leadership skills [1]. But beyond this (especially in the field of healthcare) employers are seeking caring and nurturing individuals, capable of both seeing to the medical needs at hand as well as empathizing with the patient and their individual needs [6–8].

In the following sections, we will lead you through the process of Design Thinking in the context of the student experience (Confusion, Clarity, and Completion) to give you insight and tips on how to assist your students through the Design Thinking journey, as well as some tools and exercises that we have found most valuable in our courses that you can use in class to aid in their learning throughout the Design Thinking process. Each section will be described, where relevant, in context of their:

1. Internal motivation—how they may be feeling on an individual scale
2. External standings—how they work together as a group
3. Project development—the work they are undertaking for the course

4.4.1 Confusion

The start of a Design Thinking course is undoubtedly the most confusing for the students. They must: i) [1] pivot their usual modes of learning to that of creative and innovative thinking required for Design Thinking, ii) [2] adapt to teamwork and find a balance among the members and their (very likely) different personalities, and iii) [3] personally find their value in the team and confidence in the work. It is therefore at this point that the role of the teacher is most important, to juggle these three factors and build the foundations for the students going forward.

4.4.1.1 Internal Motivation

To be able to effectively contribute, the students need to understand who they are and what they can bring to the table within their teams. The first hurdle for the teacher is to help the student understand who they are as a learner and to bring about their motivation and creativity for the tasks at hand.

Student motivation is essential for any Design Thinking process to succeed. We can argue that typically the nature of the problems we attempt to solve with the help of Design Thinking, is usually such that students will perceive them as motivating. Students are working with tangible goals trying to improve the quality of people's life, create novel innovations, or provide practical solutions for everyday healthcare work. It is easy to understand why improving health is important and that we all should have some understanding about such type of problem solving. Moreover, the human-centered approach is easily understood by the students when they perform the empathizing step. Students feel engaged because they have adopted the social, ethical, and economical values into personal interest and are willingly, and happily, acting to reach the goals of the project and produce useful outcomes.

This finding about student motivation can be examined from the theoretical perspective. It is supported by the self-determination theory, developed by Ryan and Deci [9]. It is one of the classical approaches to human motivation and personality, identifying the needs for competence, relatedness, and autonomy as basic needs to self-motivation. The theory divides different motivation types into intrinsic and extrinsic. Intrinsic motivation refers to activity, which is done because the activity itself is satisfying. The term extrinsic motivation is indicating activities which are performed to reach certain outcomes, and the extrinsic motivation can be further divided to subtypes. At one end of the extrinsic motivation spectrum, we have students performing tasks because they simply want to avoid punishments and get rewards, whereas at the other end of the spectrum, extrinsic motivation is very similar to intrinsic motivation. During the typical Design Thinking project, the students may accept the project tasks as personally important, or experience even stronger self-determination and have integrated the extrinsic values as their own values and needs.

Motivation also fuels creativity. Whether creativity can or cannot be taught remains debated, but teachers can support the learners to enhance and develop their creative thinking. Baer has summarized his and others' observations, how extrinsic

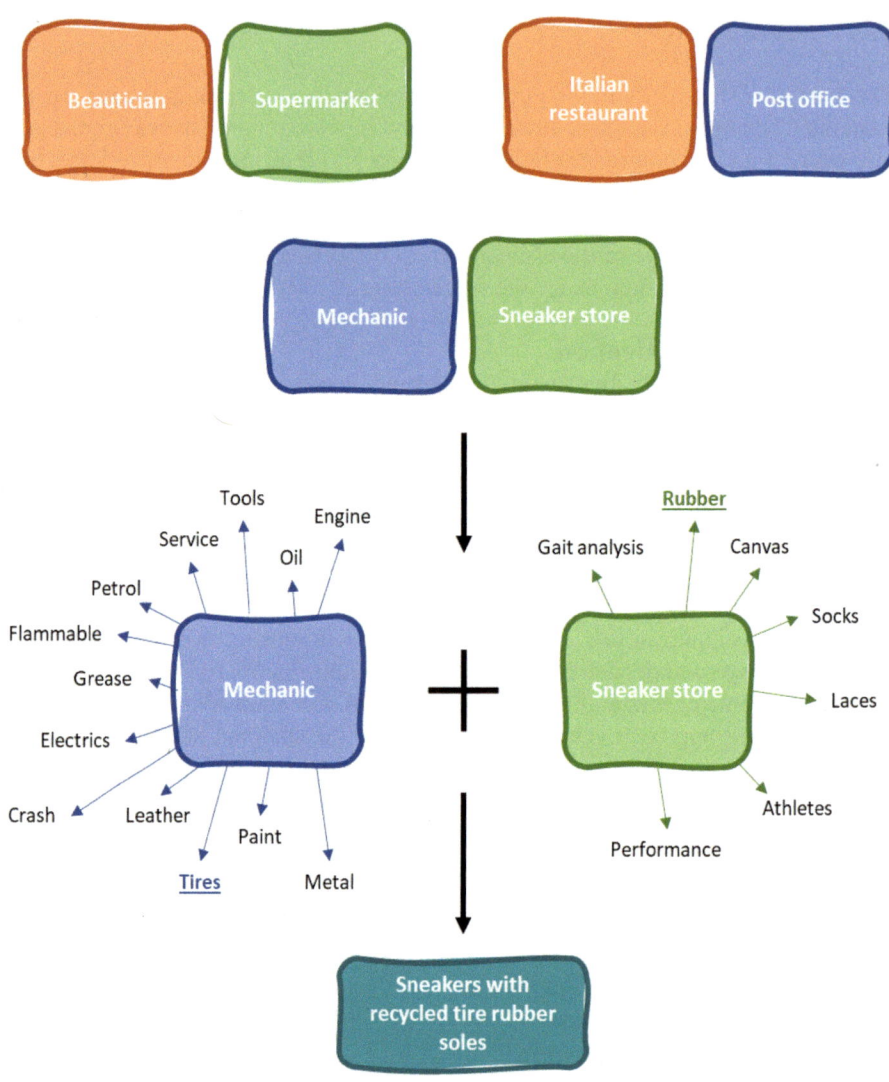

Fig. 4.2 Random Jamming involves creating a new idea from the merging of two existing ideas. In our Random Jamming exercises, the students within their group put forward either a common service or shopfront and creatively think of new products or services incorporating both. In the example provided, there are three students that have put forward two ideas each (orange, green, and blue sticky notes). The ideas put forward are mixed and randomly paired off as shown by the mixed colors. It is key that students think (or mind map) beyond the obvious for each sticky note, to push themselves into the creative space of the exercise

rewards or evaluations may negatively influence creativity, because such constraints lower intrinsic motivation [10].

A popular activity that we have implemented to kickstart student creativity is called Random Jamming (Fig. 4.2). We usually start the course with this activity as a means of an ice breaker but can be played at any point throughout the course, for example, to kickstart the ideation phase of Design Thinking. A benefit to such ice breaker activities at the start of a course is that it can also aid the teacher in the formation of groups. Such activities not only allow the students to begin building their confidence amongst their peers, but it also allows the teacher to both interact with the students to see who they are and to see how they interact with each other.

One thing to consider for student internal motivation is to understand what type of personality they possess so that they further understand themselves and their potential role within a group setting. Miller and others have used the Myers-Briggs type inventory in understanding individual personalities; and how they play into group dynamics and in the fostering of group performance, harmony, and student satisfaction (discussed further in the next section) [11]. Similarly, Isabella has implemented the Myer-Briggs personality test to instigate an individual reflection assessment for two purposes: i) to allow the students to gain new insights about themselves and what role they are best suited to play within a group; and ii) to aid the teacher in profiling the different personalities and creating dynamic groups, where possible. The journey through IEC is presented to students as the formation of a start-up. Therefore, in IEC, different Myer-Brigg personalities have been matched with the different roles commonly found within a start-up, such as CEO, CTO, COO, and so on (Table 4.3). The students can identify their role within their group and this gives them a sense of responsibility to play to.

Table 4.3 Potential Myers-Briggs type inventory (MBTI) personalities to suit common roles found in start-ups

Position	Role	Attributes	Potential MBTI
CEO: Chief Executive Officer	A jack-of-all-trades, the leader of the startup, both the team and the work at hand	Natural leader and decision maker, team player, high energy, resilient	ENTJ or ESTJ
COO: Chief Operations Officer	Works closely with the CEO to oversee the operation of the startup.	Intelligent and capable of analytical thinking and creativity, trustworthy	ISFJ or INFJ
CFO: Chief Financial Officer	The money person, needs to have a deep understanding of startup's financial capabilities through all stages	Systematic and structured habits, observant and analytical mind, efficient work ethic, responsible	INTP, ISTJ or ISTP
CTO: Chief Technology Officer	Lead technical person, focuses on the development of the technology	Ambitious, problem-solver, critical thinker, strategic	INTP or INTJ
CMO: Chief Marketing Officer	Creator of the company image. Needs to have good understanding of your market and how the product/service fits in.	Curious, observant, energetic and enthusiastic, excellent communicator, knows how to relax, very popular and friendly, artistic and innovative	ENFJ, ENTJ or ENTP
CPO: Chief Product Officer	The bridge between CTO and CMO: marries the vision of the technology being developed together with the needs of the market.		
CSO: Chief Sales Officer	The hustler of the team, turns the product/service into a flowing profit.	Confident, persistent, creative, self-motivated, enthusiastic, high energy, thrive on interaction	ESFP, ESFJ, ESTJ or ENTJ

4.4.1.2 External Standings

We will state right off the bat, that we recommend that the teacher form the student groups, instead of allowing to group themselves. Leaving this decision to the students, they will always pair off with known fellow students. Although this familiarity will benefit such individuals to boost their confidence to be creative by entering an already familiar environment, this will undoubtedly hinder the individuals that do not have already existing relationships. The teacher creating the teams allows an even playing field for all students, one in which they can grow in confidence together.

So how can we make sure the group dynamics is optimal, and everyone participates in joint activities? We have experience in facilitating international Design Thinking courses with participants from different disciplines. In an international teaching setting, it is useful to make sure that as many nationalities as possible are represented in each group. This gives the cross-cultural aspect to group work, which helps the group to understand the variety of opinions and the multiplicity of different viewpoints. Beyond this, it is important to also consider diversifying regarding gender, age, education level, study discipline, and personality (if feasible, discussed later). Such diversifications are valuable for the whole learning process, and in Design Thinking especially in the empathizing step when the students are using all the possible skills to listen to the user and trying to understand the nature of the problem. The outcome with the group of mixed nationalities may be fruitful; the end result of the Design Thinking process can be a totally surprising solution. Moreover, the cross-cultural learning experience will give a lifelong toolkit to the students for international working environments.

We have also found that the interprofessional or multidisciplinary group vitally supports the success of the Design Thinking process. For example, a design team consisting of nurses only may face problems when they try to visualize their proposed solutions or build prototypes. Students with science and especially with an engineering background are more familiar with turning their ideas into practical models to test how they function. However, in turn, they may be far less accustomed to listening to the needs of their target group. In GREAT course we also learned that students from business school can also easily help in evaluating the market value of the solutions, and those studying information technology can also shine if the proposed solution is, let's say, a mobile application. Therefore, we recommend making the groups as dynamic as possible based on the above criteria, and where feasible, target the courses for the students of a minimum of two different study programs.

As mentioned in the previous section, a mix of personalities can be beneficial to group dynamics and performance. Learning style theory gives a central role to the Thinking-Feeling and Intuition-Sensing. According to Miller and others, diversity on these two central dimensions benefits most groups [11]. Judging-Perceiving and Introversion-Extroversion dimensions affect the group harmony. They have noticed that similarities in these areas influenced student satisfaction with the course. It is easier to work in the group if the members play by the same rules. However, conflicts arising from diversity of these dimensions can induce intelligent debates and innovations which lead to enhanced group performance.

Design Thinking process should always be performed as a team effort. But how many students to a group? This may appear as a trivial question, but is in fact an important consideration for a Design Thinking course. We have found that three to four students per group is an effective number. Too few and the students may feel overwhelmed with the workload, too many and you will have mixed student contribution which will likely lead to group conflicts. Beyond this, it stimulates interprofessional and multidisciplinary collaboration, provides valuable group support, and develops creative thinking, just to mention a few obvious benefits. But the group learning also has a strong pedagogical dimension.

The active learning methods used in facilitating a Design Thinking team are often based on cooperative learning. Cooperative learning is not simply just group work, but it is defined as an instructional method, where students work together in groups to maximize their learning to reach common goals under the following conditions:

1. Positive interdependence
2. Individual accountability
3. Promotive interaction
4. Social skills
5. Group processing

This is the Johnson & Johnson model of cooperative learning [12–14], and it serves as a foundation for many active learning methods, such as problem-based learning, team-based learning, collaborative learning, and peer-assisted learning.

Positive interdependence simply means that the group members understand that they can only succeed if all the others succeed. They are linked to each other; if one fails the whole group sinks.

This interdependence naturally creates individual accountability: everyone must do their share for the group to reach the set goals. Each group member must also be able to understand all the details of the project. For promotive interaction to occur, students must provide constructive feedback, teach, and encourage each other. In order to do so, and to support the development of their social skills, they can be taught teamwork skills including leadership, decision making, and communications skills.

Instructors of the group can facilitate the learning situation to fulfill the above-mentioned conditions of cooperative learning. Felder and Brent offer several suggestions for different techniques in their review [15]. Facilitator also has a significant role in forming the team, because group learning creates its own challenges.

However sometimes, despite the best efforts of the teacher to create the most ideal groups, conflicts within groups may still arise. To mitigate potential group conflicts and to ensure that all team members understand their roles and responsibilities, team rules and policies should be agreed at the beginning of the project, and teams should be encouraged to regularly discuss and evaluate their performance and make changes if needed. To aid in this, we have previously employed the use of team charters within our courses (Fig. 4.3). Team charters are developed at the onset

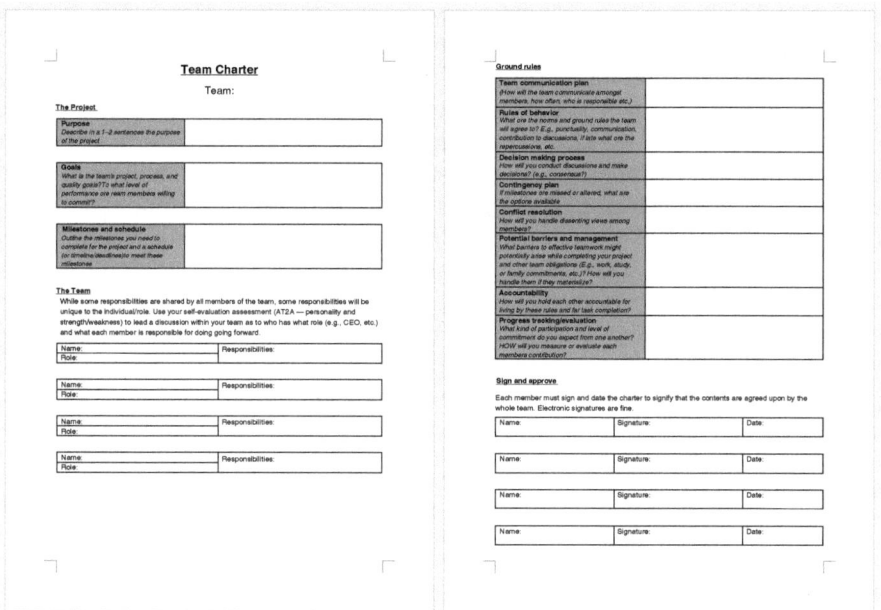

Fig. 4.3 An example template for a group chapter for students to fill in, abide by, and reflect on throughout their group work

of group formation and create a "contract" among the members to which they need to abide, and which the teachers can use to reference individual requirements later in the course, when the students' motivations might begin to slide. This idea is supported by Felder and Brent who suggest establishing team policies as a means of developing teamwork skills and dealing with uncooperative members [15].

4.4.1.3 Project Level

For participants with a background in natural science, the Design Thinking approach can certainly be very puzzling at first. Science/medicine students are not necessarily accustomed to using the maker-type of creativity in problem solving. According to Owen, "makers", or "designers", demonstrate their creativity through invention, whereas scientists are "finders", who work with discoveries, trying to find explanations [16]. Their brain is wired to look for the one and only correct answer, and in Design Thinking there is no right or wrong answer, but an almost indefinite number of better—or worse—solutions from which the "designer" will choose the best for the given situation.

To a certain extent this compares to basic scientific hypothesis testing, but usually hypotheses are built in a way that they can be proven to be simply right or wrong. Whereas in Design Thinking, the aim is to iteratively improve and prototype the initial idea toward the best possible solution. For a teacher this fundamental difference is important to understand because the teacher's role is to support the learners to endure the initial overwhelming uncertainty.

But uncertainty is good. We need to encourage students to lean into this uncertainty because this uncertainty allows for curiosity and creativity, for asking questions, and asking why. This is essential at the early stages of the Design Thinking process so that the true problem to be solved is identified. Students will often argue that they do not know enough about a topic to understand it. Our response to this is always "good!". They will likely already have some basic science or medical foundation to guide them; however, their "naivety" is advantageous for observing and analyzing a problem from a broader perspective and asking more and bigger questions. Once the questions are put forward, they can then dig for the answers to being an iterative process to gain a deeper understanding. By already starting with an in-depth understanding about a topic, they blind themselves to other opportunities and understandings of the problem and potential solutions.

We need to also ensure that ample time is spent on defining the problem. It is not a 20-min activity, but often a multi-class activity with research and discussion among team members and teachers. Our experience with both students and academics is that we have a natural tendency to jump into ideating solutions. If the problem is not properly defined, it will have a significant impact on the generation of solutions. This is especially vital in health-related problems, which are often multifaceted and complex. Without truly understanding the problem, how are we to know if we are solving the right problem? In IEC, the students are posed with a problem put forward by an academic in the field. These problems put forward are predominantly broader questions, which the students need to break down, for example, "current harbour pontoon designs are negatively impacting harbour biodiversity". If students take this problem at face value, they may fall upon a good idea, but are more likely to miss the mark and design a new pontoon that only partially solves the biodiversity issue, or not at all. Therefore, the main exercise that we employ is the "5 Whys" exercise, originally developed by founder of Toyota Industries, Sakichi Toyoda.

The 5 Whys exercise, as the name describes, is asking why to a bigger or superficial problem five times (although it does not always need to be strictly five times), until a root problem is established. The 5 Whys is a simplistic exercise in instruction. However, the 5 Whys, especially in health- or science-related problems, is not an easy activity to implement. Students will often just ask "why" to their previous statement, which may result in them looping back to a previous answer and not reaching the root problem. Instead, their "why" questions should integrate their previous answer to ensure that the why path progresses effectively. See Table 4.4 for an example of these two modes.

In healthcare, problems are often multifaceted. Encourage students to tackle their initial problem from different perspectives (for example, scientific, medical, general, economic, or environmental perspectives, etc.) to then form a "Why-tree" in which there are multiple root causes to an initial problem. Creating a Why-tree can be beneficial to put into context for the students the complexity of the initial problem and allow them to better focus on the one root problem, without trying to tackle them all. Figure 4.4 is an example of a Why-tree that we have put forward on the larger problem of hospitals being potentially hazardous places for staff. It is not a perfect Why-tree as it could have used the advice put forward above to reveal more

Table 4.4 A comparative example between a constructive versus less constructive 5 Whys activity to the complex problem of antimicrobial resistance. On the left, it is seen that a significant root cause to the rise of antimicrobial resistance is due to the lack of understanding of antibiotics and how they work, leading to mis- or over-use. By identifying this, students can then go on to ideate how they might help people understand this difficult topic, such as education programs or apps, ad campaigns, and so on. On the right, "why" is not asked in a constructive manner and so the concluding "root cause" is not in fact a root cause at all, but a symptom of antimicrobial resistance, and so no solutions can be effectively ideated

Constructive	Less constructive
Antimicrobial resistance–why is this a problem?	Antimicrobial resistance–why is this a problem?
Existing antibiotics not working	Existing antibiotics not working
Why are existing antibiotics not working?	Why is this a problem?
Antibiotics are overused	People have no way to help overcome their
Why are antibiotics overused?	infections
Doctors overprescribe antibiotics	Why is this a problem?
Why do doctors overprescribe antibiotics?	They could die.
Patients demand a solution to their infection	
regardless of the cause for the infection	
Why do they demand a solution despite the cause?	
Because they do not understand that antibiotics do not work on all infections.	

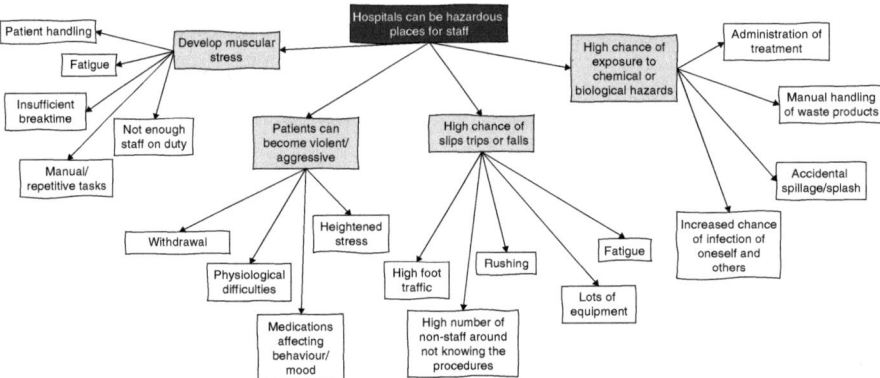

Fig. 4.4 Example of the start of a Why tree around the problem of hazards to staff in hospital settings

root causes, but there were nonetheless some interesting revelations that allowed for creative discussions and solutions. Each root could also be further elaborated on; however, we have kept it brief due to image size.

Empathy is a crucial step in the Design Thinking process, especially in healthcare. However, depending on the duration of the course, it can be difficult to implement, with limited or difficulty in accessing patients or individuals affected by the problem. If this is the case, then we strongly encourage some level of indirect modes of empathizing. This includes forums, discussion boards, or videos to gain as much

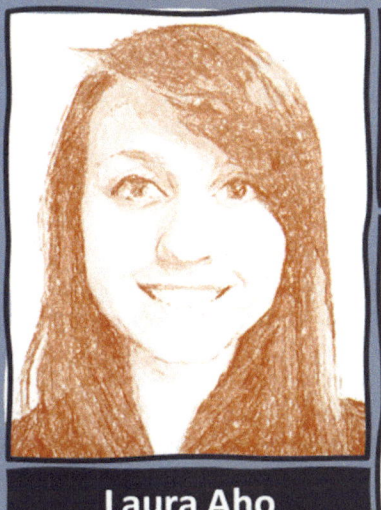

Age: 32
Location: Tampere, Finland
Occupation: Hospital nurse
Status: Married

Laura loves working as a hospital nurse, where she gets to meet people from all walks of life. At home, she loves crazy cookie Sunday's with her two young girls, creating new weird cookie combinations to bake, some a success, but most are a little questionable!

Laura Aho

Goals

- Make patients feel more comfortable to share their experiences, problems and symptoms
- Help people feel the best they can, as quickly as possible
- Create an enjoyable work environment
- Instil compassion in her kids

Frustrations

- Long tiring hours on her feet and away from her family
- Limited time with patients making it hard to create comfort and connection

Fig. 4.5 Personas are a short profile of a person of interest to you, that you can use throughout the Design Thinking person. Personas go beyond that of general demographic descriptors, but also capture emotional and behavioral observation—both directly and indirectly related to the problem at hand. Personas can be based on a certain individual or can be an amalgamation of similar personalities which you have profiled to create a fictitious individual

information as possible and bring light to factors of the problem not illuminated during the problem-defining stages. Information gathered can then be used to create fictional personas representing key persons affected by the problem (Fig. 4.5). These personas can then be used and referred to throughout the duration of the course to gain clarity and feedback on whether the problems defined, and ideas formed are truly solving the problem at hand.

4.4.2 Clarity

As the students enter ideation and allow for continued iterations of defining, empathizing, and ideating; they gain confidence in their understanding of the problem and begin to transition from confusion to clarity. It is our role then to transition to facilitators of thinking, in which we do not give answers, but instead pose questions back to the students to push and expand their thinking.

4.4.2.1 Internal Motivation and External Standings

With a strong foundation of team building built at the start of the course, team dynamics need to be continuously developed and monitored throughout the subject. Without a strong foundation, progression through the subject is significantly hindered. It is therefore vital to allow students to reflect on both their own and their team members' contributions throughout the course to understand each person's value and any shortcomings that need to be addressed. Some tensions may be visible to the teacher by observation of team interactions during class; however, there may be underlying or hidden issues unknown to the teacher. Therefore, one online tool we have utilized in complement with the team charter is called SPARKplus—a peer evaluation tool where students reflect on their own and their peers' contributions in a quantitative manner (Fig. 4.6) [17].

We have implemented this tool after each assessment to gain an understanding of student contributions and to mitigate any conflicts or lack of contribution. Because this tool gives a quantitative output of individual contributions, we have used this tool to moderate student grades to ensure that those that contribute adequately to assessments are not hindered by students that do not.

4.4.2.2 Project Development

From our observations, the first step is having a well thought-out problem question which allows for both a sense of direction for the students' thinking and the best ideas to form. Phrasing the problem as a "how might we" question pushes you into the ideation mindset. Be sure to have the team spend some time on thinking of the statement in different ways and establish a few versions of the problem statement to allow for multiple rounds of ideation. They can do this by following loosely the statement formula: "How might we (verb) (root problem)?" Have the students play around with different verbs in the statement, and where possible, see if they can bring the problem-affected population into the statement to reiterate the empathetic factor of the problem. Some examples of ways to start the statements may include:

- How might we prevent …
- How might we reduce …
- How might we aid …
- How might we determine …
- How might we identify …
- How might we improve …

CONTRIBUTION TO PROCESS/OUTPUT

1. Actively participated in activities, including class discussions and exercises, and activities outside of class organised by the team, including online communication, meetings, etc.

Student	Almost never	Seldom	Sometime	Fairly often	Almost always
Name 1	1	2	3	4	5
Name 2	1	2	3	4	5
Name 3	1	2	3	4	5
Name 4	1	2	3	4	5

2. Offered well-considered and innovative ideas and was receptive to the ideas and suggestions of other group members

Student	Almost never	Seldom	Sometime	Fairly often	Almost always
Name 1	1	2	3	4	5
Name 2	1	2	3	4	5
Name 3	1	2	3	4	5
Name 4	1	2	3	4	5

3. Contributed adequately to the overall organisation of the tasks and provided team members with required information and work within specified time-frames

Student	Almost never	Seldom	Sometime	Fairly often	Almost always
Name 1	1	2	3	4	5
Name 2	1	2	3	4	5
Name 3	1	2	3	4	5
Name 4	1	2	3	4	5

Be reflective of each team member. Use your Team Charter as a prompt of what to reflect on. Did the team member abide by the charter that they signed? What areas specifically? (min 25-max 500 words)

Student	Reflection
Name 1	
Name 2	
Name 3	
Name 4	

Fig. 4.6 Example criteria used for collecting information on peer contributions throughout the course. Students assess themselves and their peers on a scale of 1–5. They also need to write a short reflection explaining their scoring

From the Why tree about hazards to staff in hospital settings, let's take the identified problem: "increased chances of infection to oneself and others". This can be further elaborated and phrased into several "How might we..." statements to aid in brainstorming, for example, "How might we protect nurses from infectious materials?", "How might we reduce the chance of staff infecting others?", or "How might we prevent staff from becoming infected?". Although they sound similar, these slight differences in phrasing the problem can ignite different ideas and solutions.

Once a problem question/statement is established, the ideation can begin. One of the keys to effective ideation at the early stages is to not sit and ruminate on an idea for too long. Orchestrate the initial brainstorming sessions in a lighting round style, in which the students are encouraged to come up with as many ideas as possible in a short amount of time (a few minutes per round). A fun and interesting way which we have run ideation in our courses is using an exercise commonly known as 6-3-5: 6 people, 3 ideas, and 5 rounds. However, because we aim to have groups of four, we have adapted the concept into an exercise we call "Quick Rounds" (Table 4.5).

Quick Rounds is beneficial in that it allows for:

- The generation of numerous ideas
- Limited overthinking idea generation on an equal scale. That is, shy or introverted individuals are able to put their ideas forward in an equal manner to those that are more confident
- Combination or snowballing of ideas

Table 4.5 Quick Rounds is a quick and fun activity to generate several ideas in a short time. It starts with putting forward the "How might we..." question to be thought about. Then the piece of paper is passed around to each team member for 2–3 min per person. You can either do it that there is one paper for the group to be passed around, or have a separate paper per person, so that there is four papers being passed around each time set. In this latter option, you can have all four papers have the same starting question which may go down different thought paths depending on the student starting the round, or you may have four different iterations of the "How might we..." question to provoke different ideas

How might we:			
	Idea 1	Idea 2	Idea 3
Person 1	Person 1 puts down 1st idea	...2nd idea	... and 3rd idea
Person 2	Person 2 can come up with their own idea	....or snowball a previous idea	Or combine two previous ideas to create a new idea
Person 3	Person 3...		
Person 4	...and person 4 follow suit	.... Creating new ideas, snowballing or combining	...until the whole table is full of ideas to filter

Criteria	Less desirable descriptor	More desirable descriptor
How much will it cost to make?	Expensive	Cheap
Is it feasible to do?	Feasible	Impossible
Will it be difficult to do?	Difficult	Simple
Is it novel?	Exists	Innovative
Is it important to those that need it?	Negligible impact	Valuable/ beneficial/ important
Does it have room to evolve?	Specific	Broader impact

Fig. 4.7 The 2 × 2 Matrix activity is a fantastic way to filter ideas early and effectively based on their merit. Create a 2 × 2 grid with an X and Y axis. On each axis, put forward a less and more desirable descriptor of a criteria to evaluate the idea, for example, "How much would it be to make the idea?": expensive (less desirable) and cheap (more desirable). Categorize each idea based on the criteria to narrow down the ideas to pursue. If you have several ideas in the "pursue category", you can run another round of the matrix with different criteria on the axes. Some examples of criteria have been included

Once a pool of ideas has been generated, a fantastic exercise we have implemented is the "2 × 2 Matrix" as a means of filtering ideas on their potential based on established feasibility criteria such as cost, difficulty, innovation, novelty, and so on (Fig. 4.7). This activity is an effective way to filter ideas in a diplomatic manner, so as to not have the rejection of ideas be misconstrued as a reflection of the individual that put forward the idea.

Although the Design Thinking process puts forward individual stages, the actuality is that each stage bleeds into each other. That is, for example, there will always be elements of defining, empathizing, and testing during the ideation phase. This is how the best ideas are developed. It is therefore essential to encourage students to continually undergo this iterative process within the groups, but to also have formative feedback throughout the Design Thinking process, whether it is from the teachers, peers, or external mentors. As mentioned previously, our initial problems are put forward by leading academics in the respective field. We invite the mentors to attend class periodically throughout the course to provide feedback to the students, answer their questions, and validate their ideas regarding feasibility and novelty. This is especially important in science and healthcare given the complexity of the problems posed.

4.4.3 Completion

The ultimate culmination to all their hard work of the course is the showcase of their pitch. This is a very daunting task for many, and so it is our responsibility as the teacher to make this occasion as special as we can. Do not just treat it as another assessment—celebrate them. Invite the mentors and anyone else that has helped the students along the way. Wherever we could, we would bring some snacks to celebrate their hard work at the end of the pitch, where they can unwind and interact with the class and invited audience members. This small celebration from you as the teacher speaks volumes to the students, as it is a means of validation and acknowledgement of their achievements.

The pitch content will vary between courses depending on the focus and intentions of the course. We have included an example of pitch points in Table 4.6 that we use in our courses for 15–20-min pitch. However, what we would stress is that each student speaks and answers questions. This is one of the most valuable exercises the students will complete in the course, to show their understanding and contribution. Further, the structure of the pitch will vary from project to project. The layout presented below is simple one example of a pitch (Table 4.6); however, it may not be the more effective way for a group to pitch their specific idea.

An interesting question to arise while writing this chapter is whether, outside of the overall celebrations, should there be prizes for the best pitch presentations? And if so, what kind of prizes? We have debated both sides, and instead of having a clear-cut decision, we feel it comes down to the size of the prize. When BIE first began, there was a significant monetary prize for the best project, with the intention of using the funding to kickstart the scientific investigation into the hypothetical idea. Although the intent was genuine and significantly ignited the students to perform exceptionally, it resulted in significant internal fighting within the winning groups, whereby some group members attempted to bully the others out of the project and to sign over their IP rights. Ever since, prizes have been only symbolic in nature,

Table 4.6 Questions to consider when composing a pitch

Content to cover
The open
How can we hook the audience in?
The what
What is the problem?
Why is it a problem? Why should we care?
The who
Who is affected by the problem?
What is the extent of the problem? (Market analysis)
The how
How are you solving the problem—what is your solution?
How does it work? (Scientific and/or technical explanation)
How does it compare to existing alternatives and why/how is your idea better or novel? (Intellectual property)
How will it be made, for how much (cost), and how much can you make (profit)? (Production and manufacturing, financial analysis, competitor analysis)
How does it solve the problem you described?
The close
Who are you (the team)?
Why should we (the audience) join you to solve this problem with your idea?

such as certificates for all participants, with an added note of "best pitch" or "people's choice", plus a small token. This is a significantly fairer approach without burdening the students with added pressure.

4.5 Conclusion

Design Thinking is becoming an increasingly valuable tool, not just in business and IT where it has been readily implemented, but in all areas that it expands into, such as science and healthcare. Incorporation of Design Thinking into healthcare education is of significant value as it creates a heightened desire and responsibility of training healthcare workers to create healthcare experiences in which the patient and their wants and needs are the center of attention.

Implementing Design Thinking into healthcare course work is a challenging task but is ultimately rewarding both for the students and for the teachers. It allows a different sense of accomplishment, in which the students are empowered in their ability to tackle a difficult problem and bring a valuable and needed solution to the table. We have outlined in this chapter different perspectives and exercises that we have implemented in our own Design Thinking courses that we feel are of most value. But these tasks are nothing without creating the right environment for Design Thinking. So, we would like to leave you with a few final thoughts about how to create an environment that invokes thoughtfulness and creativity in our students:

- Encourage the students to fail (in their ideas), and often. And we use the word "fail" loosely, because their ideas are not failures, but opportunities for later time, or opportunities to build upon or pivot.
- Show them that it's ok to not have all the answers all the time, including the teacher. Your students will be working on a variety of complex problems, and it is not expected for you to be an expert in it all. I tell my students truthfully if I do not know something, and instead I use it as a learning opportunity for both me and the students as it opens the door for questions and ideas from everyone.
- Ensure that all ideas are heard and noted. Often quiet students may feel embarrassed or fearful to contribute, so be sure to ask them questions and have all voices heard. This will also encourage the other team members to do the same.
- Bring in external opinions, whether it be mentors, scientists, patients, and so on. Students going through this process may go down a rabbit hole of focus and may make the tasks at hand daunting and unachievable. Having the same people and same voices around them further spurs this on. Instead, inviting sporadic external influence will bring about fresh and new ideas and perspectives and will re-energize the students for the tasks.
- And finally, create a relaxed atmosphere. Remove the teacher-student barrier and instead allow for casual conversation between you and the students. By breaking down this wall, students are much more comfortable and willing to contribute to class discussions. Just have fun with it all!

References

1. Wrigley C, Straker K (2017) Design thinking pedagogy: the educational design ladder. Innov Educ Teach Int 54(4):374–385
2. Panke S (2019) Design thinking in education: perspectives, opportunities and challenges. Open Educ Stud 1(1):281–306
3. Wolcott MD, McLaughlin JE, Hubbard DK, Rider TR, Umstead K (2021) Twelve tips to stimulate creative problem-solving with design thinking. Med Teach 43(5):501–508
4. Sandars J, Goh P-S (2020) Design thinking in medical education: the key features and practical application. J Med Educ Curric Dev 7:2382120520926518
5. Madson MJ (2021) Making sense of design thinking: a primer for medical teachers. Med Teach 43(10):1115–1121
6. Beaird G, Geist M, Lewis EJ (2018) Design thinking: opportunities for application in nursing education. Nurse Educ Today 64:115–118
7. Padagas RC (2021) Design thinking in a professional nursing course – its effectiveness and unearthed lessons. Revista Romaneasca pentru Educatie Multidimensionala 13(2):132–146
8. Park M, Giap TT, Jang I, Jeong M, Kim J (2022) Listening to patients' voices: applying the design-thinking method for teaching person-centered care to nursing students. Nurs Forum 57(1):9–17
9. Ryan RM, Deci EL (2000) Self-determination theory and the facilitation of intrinsic motivation, social development, and well-being. Am Psychol 55(1):68–78
10. Baer J (2013) Teaching for creativity: domains and divergent thinking, intrinsic motivation, and evaluation. In: Gregerson MB, Kaufman JC, Snyder HT (eds) Teaching creatively and teaching creativity. New York, Springer, pp 175–181
11. Miller JE, Trimbur J, Wilkes JM (1994) Group dynamics: understanding group success and failure in collaborative learning. New Dir Teach Learn 1994(59):33–44
12. Johnson D, Johnson R (2018) Cooperative learning: the foundation for active learning. In: Active learning - beyond the future. IntechOpen, London
13. Johnson DW, Johnson RT (2009) An educational psychology success story: social interdependence theory and cooperative learning. Educ Res 38(5):365–379
14. Johnson DW, Johnson RT, Smith KA (2014) Cooperative learning: improving university instruction by basing practice on validated theory. J Excell Univ Teach 25(4):1–26
15. Felder RM, Brent R (2007) Cooperative learning. Active learning, ACS symposium series, vol 970. American Chemical Society, Washington, pp 34–53
16. Owen CL (2007) Design thinking: notes on its nature and use. Design research quarterly 2(1):16–27
17. Improving self- and peer assessment processes with technology Campus-Wide Information Systems (2009) 26(5):379–399. https://doi.org/10.1108/10650740911004804

Design Thinking Driven Solutions for Health

5

Janne Pühvel, Janne Kommusaar, and Annika Nordberg

5.1   Introduction

Design thinking methodology has been used a lot in health care during the recent years for developing patient-centered solutions. In this chapter, you will get an overview of what kind of solutions have been developed for health care using design thinking methodology during the recent years. Two examples of studies (Ector et al. [1] and Almaghaslah et al. [2]) are given in the fourth part of this chapter to illustrate the complete process. You can also find information about methods used in different studies and an overview of benefits and challenges reported by researchers.

The literature search was done in March 2022 in the following databases: Medline, Cinahl, Pubmed, Web of Science, PsycInfo, and Scopus. Search words used were "Design thinking" AND "Intervention" AND "Health*". The inclusion criteria were as follows: the research should be a case study or intervention; full-text; peer-reviewed; and published from 2020 to 2022. Forty articles were found in the databases. Duplicates were removed and studies about education were excluded because those are covered in the previous chapter of this book. After reading full text, studies where design thinking was only mentioned, but it was not explained how it was used, were excluded. The final number of studies included in this review was 15.

J. Pühvel · J. Kommusaar
Faculty of Medicine, Department of Nursing Science,
University of Tartu, Tartu, Estonia
e-mail: janne.puhvel@ut.ee; janne.kommusaar@ut.ee

A. Nordberg (✉)
Faculty of Medicine, Department of Nursing Science,
University of Turku, Turku, Finland
e-mail: anmaau@utu.fi

5.2   Overview of Health Interventions Using Design Thinking Approach

In this part, you will have a summary of the solutions created for health using the design thinking approach. Also, it is explained why and how this methodology has been combined with other methodologies.

The internet and mobile phones have become a normal part of our everyday life, and this can also be seen in the health care sector, where more and more apps and web-based solutions are designed to improve patients' lives. Mobile health (mHealth) and e-health have the potential to improve access to health care and make information exchange easier. However, not all apps and internet platforms are successfully adopted to use by the patients. Design thinking emphasizes the importance of engaging all stakeholders and therefore increases the chance of successfully implementing the product.

While developing mHealth and e-health solutions, design thinking has been used, for example, for needs assessment of an electronic cross-facility health record with the purpose to develop a prototype to improve information sharing [3]; building a national data collection and reporting system for health emergencies like the Ebola outbreak in Guinea, Liberia, and Sierra Leone [4]; developing a self-management support app for breast cancer survivors [5]; and developing a mission statement app for palliative care [6].

Design thinking has also been successfully used for other purposes than mobile or e-health. For instance, to understand how the design of maternity clinics impact and what improvements are needed for safety in Ref. [7], to improve outpatients' experiences in hospital pharmacies [2], and to develop playful strategies for fostering the well-being of pediatric cancer patients [8]. It has also been used to develop augmented reality electronic glasses prototype for older adults [9], and to develop an evidence-based model of care to support self-management for people with multi-morbid chronic obstructive pulmonary disease (COPD) [10].

Here is a short summary of one of the studies to illustrate what has been done. In their study about the design impact on safety in maternity clinics, Sherman et al. [7] were able to identify several human-centered design elements in the design of labor and delivery units. Those were cabinets, drawers, and closets in some labor and delivery rooms to meet the needs of the health professionals; an elevator that had all the supplies for the clinicians to treat the patient in labor during transportation; and a large format photo book demonstrating a woman giving birth by cesarean section, with the purpose to educate the patient and reduce her fear by better understand and anticipate the treatment and care.

Sherman et al. [7] also found some problem areas, which might affect patient safety. They focused on three areas in need of improvement: blood availability for hemorrhage management, appropriate space for neonatal resuscitation, and restocking and organization methods of equipment and supplies. Here are examples of recommended improvements for the second problem area: resuscitation equipment should be easily accessible and not block other supplies; there should be sufficient space for clinicians to surround the infant warming table to perform the resuscitation, and the resuscitation equipment and supplies should be updated.

Design thinking has also been combined with other methods like Information Systems Research (ISR) [11], Systems Thinking [12], Discrete Event Simulation (DES) [13], and Lean Six Sigma [14]. The authors justify combining methods with wanting to overcome the limitations of both approaches. For example, Dosi et al. [13] bring out that combining the DES with design thinking helps to make the DES more human-centered and the decision-making process of design thinking more data driven. And according to Farao et al. [11], ISR and design thinking complement each other, because while ISR does not specify the need of the end-users' participation during the technical development, design thinking does; design thinking has end-users' satisfaction and feedback as criteria, while ISR does not, and in ISR framework prototyping is time-consuming and costly, while in design thinking it is possible to create artifacts more quickly and with using less resources.

Here is a brief overview of how the approaches mentioned were combined with design thinking:

- The information system research has three cycles: the relevance cycle, where opportunities and problems of the application environment are identified; the rigor cycle, which provides past knowledge to ensure the research project's innovation; and the design cycle, where artifacts are designed and evaluated [15]. Farao et al. [11] used a framework where they integrated the empathize and define phase of design thinking into the relevance cycle, the test phase into the rigor cycle, and the ideate and prototype phase into the design cycle of ISR. The purpose of Farao et al. [11] study was to redesign an already existing mHealth app for reading the results of the tuberculin skin test.
- Systems Thinking is a holistic approach, where problems are solved by seeking to understand elements in a system, how they connect and interrelate over time and within the context of larger systems [16]. Shrier et al. [12] were developing an intervention implementation strategy for sexual and reproductive health intervention for young women with depression and used a system thinking tool, system mapping, in their empathize phase. This tool enabled them to identify and solve the implementation challenges.
- Dosi et al. [13] combined Discrete Event Simulation with design thinking and used four phases, which suited both approaches. Those were comprehension (seeking to understand the context), abstraction (defining and validating the simulation model), ideation (experimenting with different scenarios), and solution (test and implementation). Dosi et al. [13] were addressing the overcrowding problem in an emergency department.
- Sunder et al. [14] used Lean Six Sigma principles (Define-Measure-Analyze-Design-Verify), from a design thinking prospective to improve patients' satisfaction in a mobile hospital in India.

An overview of the aims of the studies mentioned in this part is given in Table 5.1. A longer and more thorough overview of two studies is given in part four of this chapter.

Table 5.1 Overview of studies using design thinking approach

Author(s) (year) Country	Title and aim
Almaghaslah et al. (2021) Saudi Arabia [2]	**Using design thinking principles to improve outpatients' experiences in hospital pharmacies: a case study of two hospitals in Asir region, Saudi Arabia** The aim was to improve outpatients' experiences in hospital pharmacies in two hospitals in Asir region, Saudi Arabia
Busse et al. (2021) Germany [3]	**Needs assessment for the development of an electronic cross-facility health record (ECHR) for pediatric palliative care: a design thinking approach** The aim was to capture how an electronic cross-facility health record might support, facilitate, and meet the specific needs of inpatient and outpatient pediatric palliative care professionals and to sought to develop an example ECHR as a mock-up based on these needs
Cunyarachi et al. (2020) Peru [9]	**Augmented reality electronic glasses prototype to improve vision in older adults** The aim was to design electronic glasses to help the elderly improve their vision
Dosi et al. (2021) Italy [13]	**Successful implementation of discrete event simulation: integrating design thinking and simulation approach in an emergency department** This paper concludes two previously (2019 and 2020) published articles with the preliminary results of a case study by presenting the full results, the emergency department's feedback, and the final decisions that were implemented to reduce overcrowding in an emergency department
Durski et al. (2020) Guinea, Liberia, sierra Leone [4]	**Design thinking during a health emergency: building a national data collection and reporting system** This study aimed to demonstrate how design thinking can be used during a complex emerging pathogen outbreak to solve acute and long-term challenges within the health information system
Ector et al. (2020) The Netherlands [1]	**The development of a web-based, patient-centered intervention for patients with chronic myeloid leukemia (CMyLife): design thinking development approach** The aim was to assess patients' evaluation of received information, information needs before CMyLife platform utilization, whether this information source is used correspondingly, and to predict patient factors in information perception
Farao et al. (2020) South Africa [11]	**A user-centered design framework for mHealth** The aim was to explore a combination of information systems research framework and design thinking approach for mHealth design in a developing, under-resourced context. The framework was used to re-design the tuberculous skin test reading app
Hou et al. (2020) Taiwan [5]	**The development of a Mobile health app for breast cancer self-management support in Taiwan: design thinking approach** The aim was to investigate the information needs of Taiwanese women with breast cancer to inform the development of a self-management support mHealth app

Table 5.1   (continued)

Author(s) (year) Country	Title and aim
Kamran and Dal Cin (2020) Canada [6]	**Designing a Mission statement Mobile app for palliative care: an innovation project utilizing design-thinking methodology** The aim was to develop a mobile application intervention to address the challenges related to advance care planning and improve the delivery of palliative care. A prototype of a mission statement app was developed
Salinas et al. (2020) USA [17]	**Transforming pediatric neuropsychology through video-based teleneuropsychology: an innovative private practice model pre-COVID-19** The aim was to increase accessibility to health care through the development of a video-based, pediatric teleneuropsychology (TeleNP) practice model
Sherman et al. (2020) USA [7]	**Understanding the heterogeneity of labor delivery using design thinking methodology to assess environmental factors that contribute to safety in childbirth** The aim was to understand how the design of labor and delivery units impacts safety and to identify spaces and systems where improvements are needed
Shrier et al. 2020) USA [12]	**Applying systems thinking and human-centered design to development of intervention implementation strategies: an example from adolescent health research** The aim of this project was to develop tools and strategies for addressing issues influencing momentary affect regulation–safer sex intervention (MARSSI) implementation in diverse clinic settings through clinic staff/ investigator collaboration
Sunder et al. (2020) India [14]	**Improving patients' satisfaction in a mobile hospital using Lean Six Sigma—a design-thinking intervention** The aim of this article is to explore the applicability of Lean Six Sigma in a mobile hospital. A case study is presented of improving patients' satisfaction in a mobile hospital, through reducing turnaround time
Tonetto et al. (2021) Brazil [8]	**Playful strategies to foster the well-being of pediatric cancer patients in the Brazilian unified health system: a design thinking approach** The aim was to identify how playfulness can be used as a strategy to improve the subjective well-being of pediatric cancer patients in the Brazilian unified health system
Yadav et al. (2021) Nepal [10]	**Using a co-design process to develop an integrated model of care for delivering self-management intervention to multi-morbid COPD people in rural Nepal** The aim was to develop a model of care for delivering evidence-based biomedical and psycho-social care to support self-management for people with multi-morbid chronic obstructive pulmonary disease (COPD) in rural Nepal

5.3   Methods Used for Developing Solutions for Health

Researchers and developers have used a variety of data collection and analyzes methods while applying the design thinking approach. In this part, a brief overview of the methods used in health care studies is given, categorized according to the five stages of design thinking.

The first stage, **empathize**, is for gaining an empathetic understanding of the problem [18]. Gaining empathy can start with a literature review [5], but it is also important to communicate with the end-user directly. To do so, developers have often used observations [2, 7, 10], direct engagement with the end-users [2, 11], in-depth [1], unstructured [10, 11], semi-structured [2, 13] interviews [3, 4, 7], and focus group discussions [5] to gain insight into the end-users' needs. During those observations and interviews, researchers/developers sometimes made notes [5, 7], took photographs [2, 5, 7], or filled a checklist [1]. Observations have also been used to identify workarounds to solve recurrent problems [13]. While engaging and conducting interviews or discussions, it is important to ask about the end-user needs, like Hou et al. [5] did, to fully empathize with the user.

While developing intervention implementation strategies for young women with depression, Shrier et al. [12] used system mapping in the empathize phase. This method enabled them to show how people and processes are related and how change occurs within different clinics. And Durski et al. [4] reviewed reports to build a national data collection and reporting system. Some other methods that have been used are workshops [4, 12], storytelling [2], video sessions [12], shadowing [2], benchmarking [13], and icebreaking games [5]. The icebreaking game Hou et al. [5] used while developing a mobile app for breast cancer self-management support, was a self-introduction card, where the participants had to write their name, nickname, date of diagnosis, current treatment status, and mood. This game did not only help to break the ice before the focus group discussion but also gave the investigators the opportunity to observe the participants and get information about their experiences at different stages of breast cancer treatment.

After empathy is gained, it is time to **define** the problem statement to express the end-user's core problem [18]. In this phase, researchers and developers [2, 3, 10] started analyzing the data gathered in the empathy phase. That has been done using, for example, discussion [5, 11, 12] and statistical [10] analysis, frameworks [1, 6], and affinity clustering [1]. Affinity clustering is a method where ideas are grouped and clustered into similar themes in categories [19]. More possibilities are "the 5 whys" method and creating a point of view [1]. "The 5 whys" is an iterative interrogative method to explore the cause-and-effect relationships underlying a specific problem, by asking why-questions. It can be used in all the design thinking phases but is particularly helpful when you need to understand the problem [20].

A well-known method that has also been useful for defining the problem statement is brainstorming, which several researchers and developers [4, 10, 17] have used. For example, Hou et al. [5] brainstormed by asking participants "How may we use the mHealth app to support you through your cancer fighting journey?", then writing those needs on post-it notes and grouping and prioritizing them. The identified problems can be exhibited by a needs map with met and unmet needs of the stakeholders, by the problem-evidence-opportunity tool, and through user persona, journey [13], or story [3] method. A user persona is a fictional character whose characteristics represent a realistic end-user; this enables to relate to the end-user's limitations, struggles, successes, and goals to create a personalized user experience [21]. The created fictional personas can then be used for the user journey or story method.

Ideate is the phase where generating ideas takes place and brainstorming is a useful method here too [18]. In health studies, brainstorming has been used a lot [3, 7, 10], but there are several other methods like brainstorming. For example, researchers have used the Round Robin method [12], brainwriting [2], mind-mapping [2, 10], and bodystorming [13]. Asking "how might we" questions [1], having discussions [3, 17], provocation, and storyboarding [2] have also been used for generating innovative ideas.

Here is a brief description of some of those techniques:

- During the Round Robin, one team member identifies a challenge, the next member proposes an unconventional solution, and the third member suggests a reason the solution would fail [12].
- Brainwriting is a technique where participants write down their ideas on paper and then pass the paper to another participant who will elaborate on the first person's ideas, and so forth.
- During mind-mapping, participants graphically build a web of relationships, by writing a problem statement in the middle of a paper and adding ideas that come to their minds. Later the ideas are connected by lines.
- Provocation is a lateral thinking technique which allows one to explore new realities to extreme degrees by making deliberately provocative statements.
- Storyboarding can help to bring a situation to life by developing a visual story relating to the problem, design, or solution. Storyboarding makes it possible to play with different scenarios while developing ideas.
- During bodystorming participants physically act out situations they are trying to innovate within. This can be done through physical activity or by enacting some of the problem scenarios that they are trying to solve [22].

In the end of the ideate phase, before starting prototyping, it can be helpful to organize the ideas by importance and difficulty [12] or synthesize collection of ideas into a cohesive applicable concept [10], especially if there are plenty of them. To visualize the ideas, it is possible to use sticky-notes, pictorial depictions [11], and sketching the mock-ups [4], but also the aforementioned mind-mapping and storyboarding.

The fourth phase of design thinking is **prototype**, which is an experimental phase where the aim is to identify the best possible solution for the problem found [18]. Here developers create many low-resolution [1] and low-fidelity [11] prototypes [2, 12] to solve the defined problem. Those prototypes have been physical models [7, 12], sketches, skits [7], mock-ups [3], handouts, graphic images [10], and drawings [13]. But it is also possible to prototype using storyboarding [12] or story chart to describe the patient's journey [10], role-play [12, 13], and Lego pricks [13].

After prototypes are made, it is time to **test** them. Prototyping and testing sometimes take place simultaneously, so that the prototypes can be refined, or new ones created based on the testing results. Testing may also result in redefining further problems and makes it possible to rule out alternative solutions [18]. Dosi et al. [13] had periodical meetings with the stakeholders to discuss if and how the different solutions could be implemented and so several options were left out.

Typical methods used for testing are trial [4, 5] or pilot [1] use of the prototypes, which may also be done via presentation of the prototypes [10, 13]. Testing includes asking feedback and for that, it is possible to use individual [5], semi-structured [6], or structured focus group [1] interviews; usability questionnaires [11]; observations [6, 11]; brainstorm session [10]; and "think aloud" method [11]. Kamran and Dal Cin [6], for example, plan to use the POEMS framework, where they organized their observational data under the headings "Peoples", "Objects", "Environment", "Messages", and "Services". Feedback can be gathered during workshops [10] and meetings [13] with the stakeholders.

To get a quick overview of the methods mentioned, please look at Table 5.2. Those are only a few examples of the methods that can be used and there are many more.

Table 5.2 Methods used in different design thinking phases

Phase	Possible methods
Empathize	System mapping
	In-depth, unstructured, and empathy interviews
	Structured and semi-structured interviews
	Focus group discussions
	Consultations
	Observations
	Checklists
	Field notes
	Photographs
	Shadowing
	Video sessions
	Storytelling activities
	Reviewing reports
	Literature review
	Workshops
	Ice breaker game
	Identification of workaround
	Benchmarking

Table 5.2 (continued)

Phase	Possible methods
Define	Brainstorming Discussion Affinity clustering The 5 whys Frameworks Creating a point of view Thematic analyses Statistical analyses Writing needs in post-it notes Prioritizing the needs User stories Problem-evidence-opportunity exhibits Needs mapping Process mapping Personas User journey
Ideate	Brainstorming Brainwriting Bodystorming Mind-mapping Provocation Storyboard The Round Robin method "How might we" questions Focus group and panel discussions Sticky-notes Pictorial depictions Sketching the mock-ups Organize ideas by importance and difficulty Collecting ideas into cohesive applicable concepts
Prototype	Developing low-resolution and low-fidelity prototypes: Physical models Sketches Skits Mock-ups Graphic images, drawings Handouts Lego bricks Storyboarding Story chart Role-play
Test	Trial/pilot use Presentation Workshop and meetings with stakeholders Asking feedback with: Individual, semi-structured, or structured focus group interviews Usability questionnaires Observations "Think aloud" method Brainstorm session

5.4   Examples of Using Design Thinking Approach to Develop Solutions for Health

5.4.1   Developing a Web-Based Platform for Patients with Chronic Myeloid Leukemia

Design thinking approach has been popular for developing mobile apps and web-based interventions. In Netherlands, Ector et al. [1] co-produced with patients and physicians a web-based platform CMyLife, which is meant for patients with chronic myeloid leukemia (CML). The platform aims to empower patients by providing adequate information. The project team was multidisciplinary and included patients, health care professionals, designers, developers, and a communication specialist. In the development process, Ector et al. [1] followed all the five phases of design thinking.

Empathize For understanding the end-user's needs and desires, Ector et al. [1] conducted in-depth interviews with patients and hematologists, and field observations to have an overview of the patient's journey in the health care system. A checklist was filled out during the observations. The information gathered was clustered into themes to identify connections, and stakeholder mapping was done, to identify all stakeholders.

The patient's strongest wish was to be cured of the disease. Other wishes were an insight into the disease, with more knowledge and comprehension, better support in understanding and coping with the symptoms, and improvement in the organization of care delivery. The hematologist desired to empower the patient, better insight into the patient-reported experiences and outcomes, improvement of guideline adherence, and provide care only when medically needed or when desired by the patient. During the observations, issues like long waiting times and receiving too little information regarding the prescription at the pharmacy were identified. Another bottleneck was the small role of the patients in their care process, and the lack of adequate tools to take the lead [1].

Define The gathered information was translated into a human-centered problem statement, by using tools such as affinity clustering, the 5 whys, frameworks, and creating a point of view. The problem statement was defined as "to empower patients and facilitate them to take the lead in their own care process". To achieve this goal, optimizing guideline adherence and therapy compliance are prerequisites [1].

Ideate The aim here was to use different stakeholders' perspectives to generate the broadest range of ideas. Ideating started with a team that contained at least one designer, patient, developer, and health care professional, and the ideas were then shared with the entire project team. "How might we" questions were asked to convert the gathered information into requirements of the innovation. In this manner, innovation concepts could be formed and tested on a small scale. A variety of solutions were proposed, and, in the end, the project team came up with a web-based innovation [1].

The prototype and test Phases ran partially parallel. In the prototype phase, Ector et al. [1] developed many quick-to-make and inexpensive prototypes. Those were, for example, screenshots of possible apps and websites. The prototypes were then iteratively tested by the end-users (4–6 patients) and refined by the team. The project team also had meetings with the stakeholders to identify missing information or to come up with new ideas [1].

The iterative testing of the prototypes resulted in the creation of a web-based platform called CMyLife (see my life) which refers to CML (chronic myeloid leukemia). The public website contains reliable information on the disease, treatment, other medical issues, the impact on social aspects, and a patient-tailored part with the following features:

- A forum for patients to meet each other and ask questions.
- Patients Know Best portal where patients are in control of their personal medical records.
- CMyLife module in the mobile phone app MedApp which is linked to the Patients Know Best portal in the app. This module makes it possible for the patients to rate their symptoms daily and get a weekly or monthly overview.
- Disease Activity—where the molecular marker measured is uploaded in the Patients Know Best record.
- Guideline Application is meant for visualizing the molecular marker levels and containing an easy stepwise explanation of the Dutch chronic myeloid leukemia guideline for patients in the chronic phase of the disease and reminders when it is time to be tested again.
- Reducing Hospital Visits which included features like.
  - Blood Samples drawn at home or nearby.
  - Pharmacy—MedApp's CMyLife module makes it possible to request a delivery of prescriptions.
  - Screen-to-Screen Consulting with the hematologists [1].

Eventually, a pilot test was run and during it, focus group interviews with patients and hematologists were conducted to gather feedback. Patients were satisfied with the screen-to-screen consultations, having blood samples drawn at home, and insights into individual laboratory results together with guidelines. The feedback on the possibility to register symptoms and medication intake varied because not all patients could imagine this to be beneficial to their management. Although the hematologists could see the value for the patients, they were still reluctant toward the platform because of the extra work and time it takes. They also pointed out a concern with the growing development of mobile interventions which are specified to one disease and the need for a universal solution [1].

5.4.2   Using Design Thinking Principles to Improve Outpatients' Experiences in Hospital Pharmacies

Another example of a design thinking driven solution is the study of Almaghaslah et al. [2], who used the design thinking approach while trying to improve outpatients' experiences in two hospital pharmacies in Saudi Arabia. In their study, they followed the five stages of design thinking to overcome the problems that were affecting the patient's experience.

Empathize   In the first stage, Almaghaslah et al. [2] interacted with patients in two hospitals to understand the user's needs, values, and desires. The research team used shadowing and observation as methods to examine users' behavior when they visited the pharmacy and used their services. They engaged with the users and had several one-to-one semi-structured interviews. In this stage researchers took pictures of the waiting areas and hospital pharmacies. Storytelling activities were also used. After these methods, a list of key problems was identified.

Define   After the data was gathered from the users, the researchers defined the problem in two steps. At this second stage, the research team tried to tackle the situation first by identifying the core problems by utilizing the collected data, and secondly by identifying the possible solutions for the users' problems. Main goal at this point was to generate as many solutions as possible to solve these problems [2].

During the empathy and define phase following problems were identified:

- Lack of comfortable environment in the pharmacies' waiting areas.
- Lack of a queue management system.
- Lack of equity in waiting times between the two genders.
- Workflow inefficiencies through ordering and supplies.

Ideate   In the third part the research team pursued creativity. Brainstorming, prototyping sessions with new techniques that included brainwriting, storyboard, mindmapping, and provocation were used for inspiration and to boost creativity [2].

Prototype   When the information was collected, the problems identified, and solutions shaped to match the user's needs, the research team started to sketch and build the prototypes. In this stage the prototypes were named to answer a specific problem [2].

In the ideate and prototype phase these solutions were developed [2]:

- Electronic-prescribing initiatives for physicians to communicate with the pharmacy.
- A queue management system.
- Redesigned waiting areas and more seats for female patients.

- More adaptive arrangements for patients with disabilities.
- Vending machines.
- Children's corner in the waiting room.
- TV screens in the waiting room.
- Bright colors in the waiting room instead of dark.
- Partitions at the end of the counter.

Test Almaghaslah et al. [2] monitored the use of the prototypes, collected feedback, and observed the users in the test stage of design thinking process. The final prototype was a model design that overcomes all the shortcomings in both hospitals.

5.5 Benefits and Challenges of Design Thinking Approach in Health Interventions

Design thinking approach can provide innovative solutions when wanting to improve the patient experience. The process considers the possibilities of multidisciplinary work and exploits them [2]. Design thinking approach enables to gain valuable insights from end-users with their life experiences and knowledge [23]. Therefore, it is easier to focus on the user's needs and prioritize the reframing of the problem before the solution is made compared to many other methods and frameworks. Design thinking approach ensures that the solution answers to the right problem and needs, and that all the stakeholders are pleased and satisfied with the result. It has been found to be a successful method in bringing together the end-users, policymakers, implementers, and researchers [10] and developing culture-sensitive solutions [2, 5].

Although involving all the stakeholders is a strength of this method, it can also be quite challenging. Some authors described having difficulties in scheduling a time suitable for everyone [5, 10, 12]. It is possible to form several small groups like Hou et al. [5] did, which may be helpful for finding meeting times and ensuring that all participants have the possibility to voice their opinion. It can also be challenging to engage patients from the marginalized community [10] and transportation too can become a problem [5] if participants from different regions are involved. The diversity of the participants also results in a wide range of views and interview conversations can sometimes be abstract. Because of that, it may be difficult to transform a wide range of users' wishes into specific needs [3].

Design thinking is beneficial for creating a diversity of prototypes and the process helps to stimulate creativity [11]. Although this approach is effective, one of the disadvantages is that it lacks a strong data-driven decision-making process [13]. The design thinking methodology is time-consuming and it's challenging to find enough time to iterate the prototypes and test the solutions [12]. At the same time the process may lead service users and providers to expect that the solution will be implemented soon after the development process and it will immediately meet end-users' needs in every way [10]. Therefore, it is important to identify the potential funding in the early process and involve funders in creating, testing, and sustaining the developed solution [10, 12].

Despite the challenges of design thinking method, the benefits are bigger, and all the authors were satisfied with the chosen methodology. The Design Thinking methodology provides an opportunity for patients and clinicians to share their experiences and problems, which helps to develop best solutions to fit the needs of patients instead of using pre-determined ideas to improve health care services [10]. The method is focused on people and solves the real problems that real people have. It allows the solution to be adapted and modified according to the needs of the end-user so that good results are obtained [9]. Involving all the stakeholders in the development process also helps to reduce the challenges in implementing the final product [11].

References

1. Ector GICG, Westerweel PE, Hermens RPMG, Braspenning KAE, Heeren BCM, Vinck OMF, de Jong JJM, Janssen JJWM, Blijlevens NMA (2020) The development of a web-based, patient-centered intervention for patients with chronic myeloid leukemia (CMyLife): design thinking development approach. J Med Internet Res 22. https://doi.org/10.2196/15895
2. Almaghaslah D, Alsayari A, Alyahya SA, Alshehri R, Alqadi K, Alasmari S (2021) Using design thinking principles to improve outpatients' experiences in hospital pharmacies: a case study of two hospitals in Asir region, Saudi Arabia. Healthcare 9. https://doi.org/10.3390/healthcare9070854
3. Busse TS, Jux C, Kernebeck S, Dreier LA, Meyer D, Zenz D, Zernikow B, Ehlers JP (2021) Needs assessment for the development of an electronic cross-facility health record (Echr) for pediatric palliative care: a design thinking approach. Children 8. https://doi.org/10.3390/children8070602
4. Durski KN, Singaravelu S, Naidoo D, Djingarey MH, Fall IS, Yahaya AA, Aylward B, Osterholm M, Formenty P (2020) Design thinking during a health emergency: building a national data collection and reporting system. BMC Public Health 20:1896. https://doi.org/10.1186/s12889-020-10006-x
5. Hou IC, Lan MF, Shen SH et al (2020) The development of a mobile health app for breast cancer self-management support in Taiwan: design thinking approach. JMIR Mhealth Uhealth 8:e15780. https://doi.org/10.2196/15780
6. Kamran R, Dal Cin A (2020) Designing a Mission statement Mobile app for palliative care: an innovation project utilizing design-thinking methodology. BMC Palliat Care 19:151. https://doi.org/10.1186/s12904-020-00659-1
7. Sherman JP, Hedli LC, Kristensen-Cabrera AI, Lipman SS, Schwandt D, Lee HC, Sie L, Halamek LP, Austin NS (2020) Understanding the heterogeneity of labor and delivery units: using design thinking methodology to assess environmental factors that contribute to safety in childbirth. Am J Perinatol 37:638. https://doi.org/10.1055/s-0039-1685494
8. Tonetto LM, da Rosa VM, Brust-Renck P, Denham M, da Rosa PM, Zimring C, Albanti I, Lehmann L (2021) Playful strategies to foster the Well-being of pediatric cancer patients in the Brazilian unified health system: a design thinking approach. BMC Health Serv Res 21:985. https://doi.org/10.1186/s12913-021-07018-7
9. Cunyarachi LO, Santisteban AS, Andrade-Arenas L (2020) Augmented reality electronic glasses prototype to improve vision in older adults. Int J Adv Comput Sci Appl 11. https://doi.org/10.14569/IJACSA.2020.0111185
10. Yadav UN, Lloyd J, Baral KP, Bhatta N, Mehta S, Harris MF (2021) Using a co-design process to develop an integrated model of care for delivering self-management intervention to multi-morbid COPD people in rural Nepal. Heal Res Policy Syst 19. https://doi.org/10.1186/s12961-020-00664-z

11. Farao J, Malila B, Conrad N, Mutsvangwa T, Rangaka MX, Douglas TS (2020) A user-centred design framework for mHealth. PLoS One 15:e0237910. https://doi.org/10.1371/journal.pone.0237910
12. Shrier LA, Burke PJ, Jonestrask C, Katz-Wise SL (2020) Applying systems thinking and human-centered design to development of intervention implementation strategies: an example from adolescent health research. J Public Health Res 9. https://doi.org/10.4081/jphr.2020.1746
13. Dosi C, Iori M, Kramer A, Vignoli M (2021) Successful implementation of discrete event simulation: integrating design thinking and simulation approach in an emergency department. Prod Plan Control:1. https://doi.org/10.1080/09537287.2021.1996651
14. Sunder MV, Mahalingam S, Krishna MSN (2019) Improving patients' satisfaction in a mobile hospital using Lean Six Sigma—a design-thinking intervention. Prod Plan Control 31:512–526. https://doi.org/10.1080/0953728720191654628
15. Hevner A (2007) A three cycle view of design science research U-CARE view project modeling customer churn view project. Scand J Inf Syst 19
16. What is systems thinking?—Definition from WhatIs.com. https://www.techtarget.com/searchcio/definition/systems-thinking. Accessed 20 Oct 2022.
17. Salinas CM, Bordes Edgar V, Berrios Siervo G, Bender HA (2020) Transforming pediatric neuropsychology through video-based teleneuropsychology: an innovative private practice model pre-COVID-19. Arch Clin Neuropsychol 35:1189. https://doi.org/10.1093/arclin/acaa101
18. What is design thinking? | Interaction Design Foundation (IxDF). https://www.interaction-design.org/literature/topics/design-thinking. Accessed 20 Oct 2022.
19. Design thinking and affinity mapping | Design & innovation global. https://www.designinnovationglobal.com/design-thinking/articles/design-thinking-and-affinity-mapping. Accessed 20 Oct 2022.
20. What are 5 whys? | Interaction Design Foundation (IxDF). https://www.interaction-design.org/literature/topics/5-whys. Accessed 20 Oct 2022.
21. User Personas: What are they and why they matter in UX design. https://www.wix.com/blog/creative/2020/02/how-to-create-a-user-persona-ux/?utm_source=google&utm_medium=cpc&utm_campaign=16242205830%5E136002928760&experiment_id=%5E%5E582527080077%5E%5E_DSA&gclid=CjwKCAjwyryUBhBSEiwAGN5OCBNf7WBC3wLk48c39HzVK0K40q7zQAghU8nVqmTEtlWp6h_sS9MzxBoCNFUQAvD_BwE. Accessed 20 Oct 2022.
22. Introduction to the essential ideation techniques which are the heart of design thinking | Interaction Design Foundation (IxDF). https://www.interaction-design.org/literature/article/introduction-to-the-essential-ideation-techniques-which-are-the-heart-of-design-thinking. Accessed 20 Oct 2022.
23. Doley JR, McLean SA, Griffiths S, Yager Z (2021) Designing body image and eating disorder prevention programs for boys and men: theoretical, practical, and logistical considerations from boys, parents, teachers, and experts. Psychol Men Masculinity 22:124. https://doi.org/10.1037/men0000263

Using Design Thinking in Nursing Management and Leadership

6

Eriikka Siirala, Outi Tuominen, and Sanna Salanterä

6.1 Self-management to Support Nursing Management and Leadership

Nurse managers work under constant pressure as both implementers of requirements from the strategic level and leaders of nurses providing clinical care [1, 2]. The main tasks of nursing leadership are planning, implementing, and evaluating departmental activities [3]. In this role, the nurse manager and leader contributes as a role model who sets goals for the department, supports the nursing staff, is approachable, and remembers to take care of her/his own well-being. The work is autonomous and requires the ability to schedule one's own tasks to achieve objectives [4–6].

Self-management is emphasized in the workplace to ensure a balanced leadership approach. Classically, self-management refers to how a nursing leader manages and schedules the planning, implementation, and evaluation of nursing activities, and how she or he monitors the achievement of goals. Self-management is a conscious effort to direct one's own actions and thinking [7] to achieve things that are meaningful to oneself and others. It is said that self-management is about

E. Siirala (✉)
Innovation Centre, The wellbeing services county of Southwest Finland and Faculty of Medicine, University of Turku, Turku, Finland
e-mail: Eriikka.siirala@varha.fi

O. Tuominen
Department of Paediatrics and Adolescent Medicine, Turku University Hospital and Faculty of Medicine, Department of Nursing Science, University of Turku, Turku, Finland
e-mail: outi.tuominen@tyks.fi

S. Salanterä
Faculty of Medicine, Department of Nursing Science, University of Turku and Turku University Hospital, Turku, Finland
e-mail: sansala@utu.fi

influencing oneself and others. In doing so, it has been found that job satisfaction and dedication to work and job performance improve, and possibly absenteeism decreases. This also leaves room for creativity, which is needed at work.

Research has approached at self-management from different perspectives and self-management is one of the key skills for the future of work. The Future of Jobs Report (2020) [8] by the World Economic Forum (WEF) highlights key self-management skills such as active learning, the ability to cope with stress and uncertainty, the ability to manage different work tasks, or the ability to be flexible. Stress tolerance can be improved by prioritizing important tasks and planning work. In addition, taking care of well-being and recovery is necessary to balance work life with one's personal daily life [8].

Self-management is needed due to the constant rush, the change in the nursing environment, and the resulting prioritization of work. In prioritizing work, the nurse manager must be aware of the responsibilities and duties of his/her own managerial role. The nurse manager must be aware of what is essential, important, and useful in the work. The order of his or her tasks is hardly predetermined, so she or he must be able to prioritize them. The manager must also be able to identify his or her own weaknesses and strengths and take them into account when planning and achieving her own objectives. Good self-management enables creative action, motivates self and others, and contributes to the achievement of goals [9]. It helps and supports the nurse manager to adapt to changing and uncertain situations.

6.2 Nursing Management and Leadership in VUCA Environment

The nursing management and leadership environment can be described through the phenomena of *volatility, uncertainty, complexity, and ambiguity*. This type of environment is referred to as a VUCA environment, also referred to as a VUCA phenomenon [10]. The acronym describes the current unpredictable world situation, which emphasizes the constant change, uncertainty, and ambiguity of the environment on the one hand, and the individual's ability to change, tolerate uncertainty, and endure change, on the other.

The VUCA environment has been highlighted as a phenomenon for several years. The theory described changes that happened very fast, and it has been first used in 1987 by Warren Bennis and Burt Nanus leadership theory. It is driven by several mega-trends that are changing society on a large scale, such as globalization and digitalization. Recent global crises such as pandemics have reinforced the phenomenon [11, 12]. The problems brought about by the VUCA phenomenon in nursing may lead to a situation of the nurse manager where managing work and workload and maintaining time schedules are difficult and have a negative impact on well-being [13].

The VUCA phenomenon has been used particularly in crisis management [11]. The VUCA phenomenon can also be considered in the concrete context of nursing.

The challenges faced in day-to-day nursing management and leadership are complex and the solutions are not always unambiguous [14]. Such problems may include instability in human resources, uncertainty about changes in patient well-being, the complexity of multidisciplinary teams, and sometimes ambiguity due to the ambiguity of work tasks.

Nursing management and leadership is *volatile*. Volatility is caused by changes in society, such as service system reform [11]. Nurse managers and leaders must balance existing finite resources, ever-increasing needs and change caused by surprising factors, for example. The instability caused by the surrounding society can manifest itself in the nursing profession in the *uncertainty* of how to maintain a person's ability to work and well-being at work. Nursing is constantly exposed to changes in patients' conditions, which requires management and leadership to be able to adapt to changing situations and to cope with uncertainty [14]. Changes in the unpredictable work environment are perceived as a challenge for management, because what has been experienced in the past cannot be used to manage future situations. In the future, digitalization, artificial intelligence, and technology will bring new possibilities for patient care and nursing, but they will require a renewal of operating methods and a change in operating culture. Poorly managed change creates uncertainty. Nurse managers and leaders need skills in implementing change.

The nursing environment is often described as *complex*. Complexity can refer, for example, to the rapid growth of technology mentioned above and the new solutions it brings [11]. These changes can be confusing and cause chaos. In nursing management and leadership, complexity is reflected in the increased use of technology in patient care. On the other hand, the complexity of day-to-day management is caused by multiple professional groups and different specialties working on the same unit at the same time. Responsibilities and duties vary from one professional group to another, which means that the head of nursing needs to have knowledge of multidisciplinary and how to coordinate the various players and their objectives [15]. Also, many nursing functions are interdependent, so that complexity can manifest itself precisely in the form of mutual confusion.

The work of a nurse manager and leader can be said to be *ambiguous*. Ambiguity can be broadly defined as the imprecision of information produced by multiple sources of information, where it is difficult to verify the accuracy of it [11]. In units where acutely ill patients are treated, nursing management is hectic and there is little time for the information needed for decision-making and it is not always possible to check the accuracy of the information to support decision-making [16]. Technology has brought a number of solutions to support action, but the overall picture of nursing management and leadership is not available.

The ability to adapt and accept constant change and uncertainty is needed in nursing management and leadership. Recently, it has been suggested that design thinking in self-management could support leadership in a VUCA environment [10, 17]. The method offers a novel approach to addressing challenges in nursing leadership [18].

6.3   Design Thinking Method to Support the Nurse Manager and Leader

Design thinking aims to innovate something new, such as developing a method, service, or product from an idea into a new solution. The ability to innovate is also a competitive asset for an organization. In developing new services and products, design thinking can be used both in nursing management and leadership and in the care of individual patients [6, 18–20]. Solutions developed using the methods have been shown to have a positive impact on care [19]. It has been found that design thinking provides a new tool for the development of nursing [19, 21] and self-management in a VUCA environment. The connection with Stanford design thinking method and VUCA is presented in Fig. 6.1. In the figure, it is possible to see what the VUCA phenomenon means in a nursing management and leadership environment.

Using the design thinking approach, nurse manager and leader can develop his or her own strengths and weaknesses. She plays a key role in creating a culture of creativity in the department, where design thinking serves as an excellent tool for problem solving [6]. The specificities of the VUCA climate for nursing management and leadership outlined above can also be related to supporting one's own thinking about self-management and how to succeed in it. In this kappa, design thinking is seen as a cognitive process for the nursing leader [20].

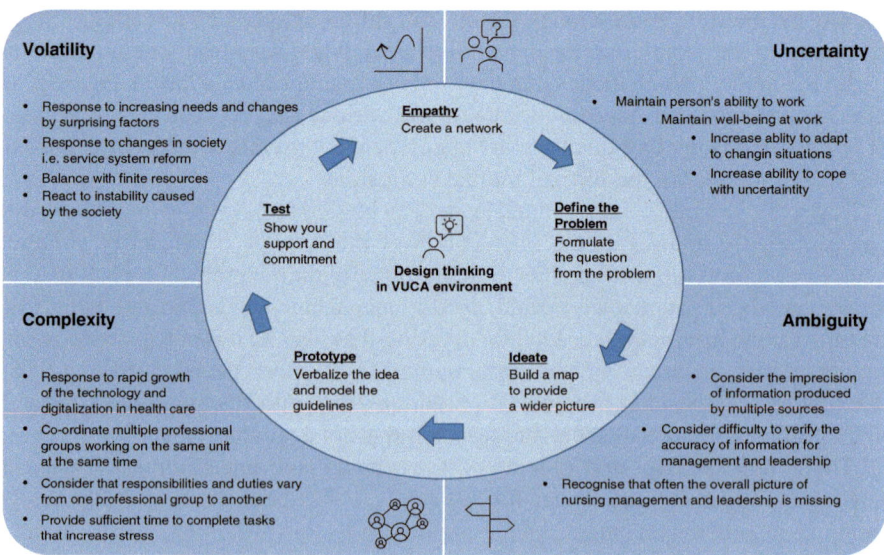

Fig. 6.1 Using design thinking in nursing management and leadership in VUCA environment

6.3.1   Empathy

The empathy stage focuses on understanding the experiences and perceptions of others about the challenge to be solved. Empathy is an important management and leadership skill that refers to a genuine caring, attitude, and acceptance of others' perspectives [22]. In the empathy stage, it is essential to put oneself in the other person's shoes in understanding the management and leadership challenge at hand [18]. One should be able to put aside one's own views while listening to the views of others on the challenge or everyday problem at hand. The key is to let go of one's own previous perceptions and be open to different ideas and views. The best way to understand the problem at hand is to interview others and, if possible, to create a picture of the environment in which the problem occurs.

The nurse managers and leaders often work alone in the unit and peer support may not be available. They should therefore create a network around them that can be used to understand different types of challenges and define the problem [6, 23]. Nursing problems are rarely limited to one specialty or professional group, so the network should include experts from as many areas as possible [18].

6.3.2   Defining the Problem

The next step is for the nurse manager and leader to define a key leadership problem from the challenge identified through empathy. The challenges and problems in the VUCA environment are often vague and difficult to delineate; the defining the problem stage requires analysis and interpretation of the information gathered in the first empathy stage. To support the analysis, the problem can be considered through questions such as "Who", "What", "Why", "Where", "When", and "How", followed by building questions around the challenge or problem to be addressed. It can be easier to identify the "yes" and the big picture when the problem is defined in the form of a question. The result of the definition is a problem statement.

6.3.3   Ideate

A problem stated in the form of a question is solved by brainstorming as many different solutions as possible. Ideating is about quality rather than quantity, as several ideas can generate new ideas, which are already slightly better, and hence solutions. The nurse manager and leader needs to be creative and unconventional, to challenge the basic solutions, and to be open to completely new solutions by thinking out of the box.

Ideation is often supported by brainstorming, where all ideas are written down on a concept map to help select the best solution. A concept map is a visual representation of ideas and solutions generated through empathy and possibly research. The map can be used to support discussion or to explain ideas. Ideation can be facilitated using supporting questions such as "how might we...". Ideas presented should not be criticized but further questions to clarify the idea should be asked. Finally, the ideas are grouped together where they are similar, and the ideas are named. The aim of the workshop is to produce as much material as possible for prototyping.

The idea map can also be used to demonstrate to other nurse managers and leaders that individual problems and challenges are part of a wider picture that is being addressed. The map not only serves as a tool for finding a solution but also supports the development of personal thinking and empathic skills.

6.3.4 Prototype

Prototype refers to the first solution that could be feasible from an ideation point of view and which is then implemented. The aim is to describe the developed idea with as little work as possible, but still in line with the intended use. In the prototyping phase, the nurse manager and leader must accept that the solution developed may not be as expected, in which case the challenge-solving process and ideation needs to be redirected and possible other ideas used, or the empathy phase restarted. If necessary, the prototyping phase will also include a preliminary cost analysis.

In nursing management and leadership, a verbal description can serve as an example of a prototype to be tested in the final phase of design thinking. The description can be a model or a guideline to see how the idea works and how it could be further developed.

6.3.5 Test

In the test phase, the prototype developed in nurse management and leadership is tested in everyday nursing practice, in real management situations. The feedback from the working team helps to improve and further develop the solution, which also improves the quality of the solution. What is required from the working community is cultural sensitivity and an open environment that allows for the testing of new solutions and the potential for change that this entails.

The support of the nurse manager and leader in the work community is essential to ensure that staff are also committed to the implementation of the new solution [24].

6.4 Case Example of an Innovation in Nursing Management and Leadership Implemented Using Design Thinking

The case example in nursing management and leadership is based on Outi Tuominen's dissertation published in 2020. The innovation called Respa © is widely used in Finnish hospitals.

6.4.1 Empathy as the Starting Point and Defining the Problem

The Children and Adolescent Division is responsible for specialized care for children and adolescent at Turku University Hospital. It has more than 300 nursing staff, including 18 float pool nurses. These nurses were designated to continually change units. In addition, organization used permanent nursing staff to "float" from their regular ward to other areas, a practice known as "floating shifts". This may be required in the case of sudden staff absence due to sickness or as a temporary alternative to booking substitute nurses [25]. In addition to float pool nurses, floating nurse reserve staff and loan staff were used in our domain. This equalizes staffing levels and workloads in the units. The practice is often driven by employer need rather than by the voluntary nature of the nurses [26]. The need for extra nurses was explored by email, telephone, messages, and meetings. This took up a huge amount of the time of the nurse managers and nursing supervisors [27].

In the past, float pool nurses' shifts were printed out in six-week cycles as a basic for the units' nurse managers and leaders. In practice, this meant that float pool nurses were already booked two days after the lists were published. The paper rosters were difficult to interpret, and float pool nurses were not used for what they were intended, that is, to cover sudden absences. The picture of the paper-based system of float pool nurses is presented in Fig. 6.2. In addition, organization used permanent nursing staff to "float" from their regular ward to other areas, a practice known as "floating shifts" [28].

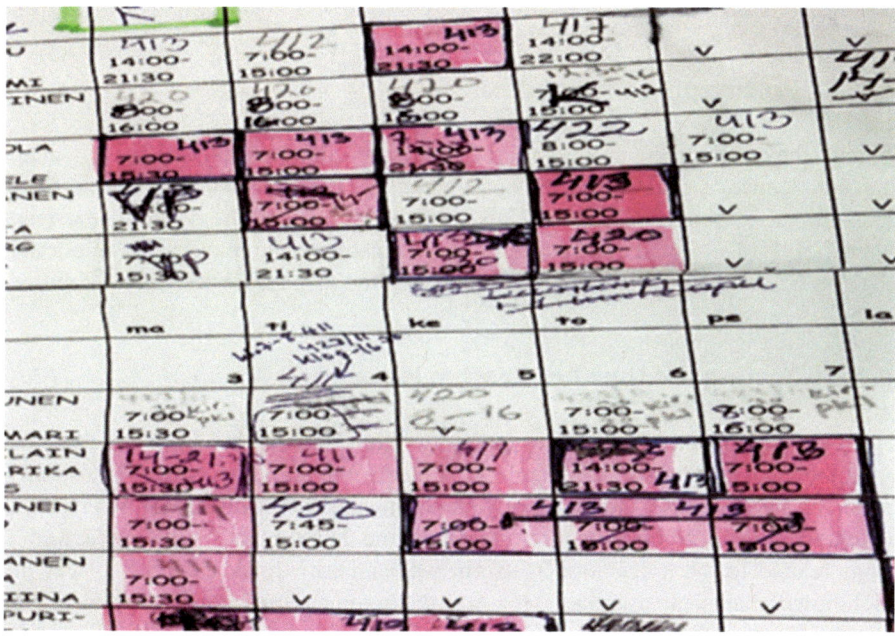

Fig. 6.2 Printed scheduling list (paper-based system) of float pool nurses

The problem had been identified, back-up staffing needed to be made available to meet the sudden need, and coordination of nurse manager of float pool nurses needed to be streamlined. Previous studies showed that similar groups of nursing staff could also be managed using electronic applications. In Finland, no equivalent system was available.

6.4.2 Ideating the Solutions

Ideating started with something as simple as a roster of floating nurses' shift and stored it electronically for use by nurse managers and leaders instead of printed scheduling list. There was also a need to add available floating nurses in to it, so that this information is automatically available to everyone.

As the idea evolved at the idea level, it became clear that the app needed to be also available to nursing staff outside of office hours and should be easily integrated into the organization's HR systems, particularly into the shift scheduling system, that has been used to schedule float pool nurses' shifts in a 3-week rotation. It should enable the reservation of floating nurses and float pool nurses in the same view and provide open data about the scheduling of float pool nurses and rescheduling of floating nurses [25].

In addition, the app should enable communication about staffing needs. The app included options for book float pool nurses, add and book floating nurses, add request for additional nursing staff needs by units and for nursing staff, option to add their willingness to work extra shifts.

6.4.3 Prototyping the Solution

Finally, the development process was carried out in collaboration with nurse managers and leaders from the pilot departments of Turku University Hospital, the Department of Nursing Science (University of Turku) and the development manager from Fujitsu Finland. The role of nurse managers and leaders was important; they proposed ideas for creating and modifying the IT-based rescheduling solution.

6.4.4 Testing the New Application Innovation Respa©

Bringing the application to the testing phase required time and close collaboration with the application developer. In the first phase, the app was tested in a test environment. In this phase, corrected private points and added functionalities (such as colors to indicate the booking reasons) were done. During this testing phase, limitations related to the application platform were identified; for example, it was not web-based, that is, the user had to log in to the organization's computer to access the system. There we also need to split float pool nurses' shift, for some cases were they change unit between the shift.

Once the first operationally acceptable version was ready, it was given to the nurse managers and leaders for test use. Based on the feedback received, the application was further developed and finally the fourth version was unanimously approved for use.

In the first phase, we tested the mini application alone in a test environment. In this phase, we corrected private points and added functionalities (such as colors to indicate the booking size). During this testing phase, we also identified limitations related to the application platform; for example, it was not web-based, that is, the user had to log in to the organization's computer to access the system. We also had to find a solution to the problem that a deputy's shift could be split between two different units.

Once the first operationally acceptable version was ready, it was given to the nurse managers and leaders for test use. Based on the feedback received, the application was further developed and finally the fourth version was unanimously approved for use.

6.4.5   Implementing the Innovation

The implementation of the application in organization domain was surprisingly smooth. This is certainly related to the fact that this problem had been waiting for a solution for a long time. The fact that nurse managers and leaders were involved in the development of the application certainly facilitated the implementation [29].

An initial challenge was that the transition to the application was sometimes slow. Nurse managers and leaders did not fully trust the new application and continued to send emails and call each other. This was quickly recognized and it was found that although the app works and is easy to use, it needed a set of rules that everyone would follow [30]. Nurse managers and leaders need mutually agreed shared policies to guide decision-making, regarding the allocation of floating nurses to build trust in the system functionality [30].

The nursing staff implemented the system smoothly. They now had visibility of the available float pool and floating nurses in a whole new way. On the other hand, at the same time, it became clear that they also needed agreed shared policies for when units should release a floating nurse into the system.

Alongside the development of a single application, organizations must remember that changing the way that has always worked need to be evaluated afterward. Gathering feedback on the usability of the application through a usability study is recommended, as is evaluating the change in approach in relation to staff experience. The development process of the IT-based staffing solution is presented in Table 6.1

Table 6.1 IT-based staffing solution development

IT-based staffing solution development	**Timeline** The delepment process took six months, including the piloting phase. Third version were accepted in the daily use.
	Software The solution for the scheduling and rescheduling float pool nurses and floating nurses contains a Microsoft SQL server, a databased management method with the central function of storing and retrieving the data.
	Stored data The solution contained the following data: Reasons for sudden abcenses of nursing staff, number of booked floating shift, number of unstaffed shifts and number of staff employed as temporaty staff outside the organisation.
	The recearcher role Interwieving, motivating nurse managers, collecting feedback during the develpoment process and provide educationg for the end users
	Nurse managers role The development process were carried out with close colloboration with nurse managers, they proposed ideas for modifying platform.
	Research Nurse managers work task were studied before and after the implementation as well as usability of the solution. Nursing staff experience about floating shifts were studied in percpective of exprience of stress
	Access Open access for the end users was the main principle during the development process

6.4.6 What Does Design Thinking Teach in the Context of Management and Leadership?

Creating something new requires courage and the ability to look at things from a new perspective and in a new way. In this development, one employee's idea was enriched by enabling the actors to participate in the development of the application. Development work and new creation require cooperation skills and especially communication skills, so that the change can also be implemented in the operating environment. If a single employee does not have these skills, it is worth building a team where the skills of different people support the completion of the idea.

References

1. Pegram AM, Grainger M, Sigsworth J (2014) Strengthening the role of the ward managers: a review of the literature. J Nurs Manag 22(6):685–696. https://doi.org/10.1111/jonm.12047
2. Zhu M, Yang Z, Liang X, Lu X, Sahota G, Liu R, Yi L (2016) Managerial decision-making for daily case allocation scheduling and the impact on perioperative quality assurance. Transl Perioper Pain Med 1(4):20–30

3. Miller A, Weinger MB, Buerhaus P, Dietrich MS (2010) Care coordination in intensive care units: communicating across information spaces. Hum Factors 52(2):147–161. https://doi.org/10.1177/0018720810369149
4. Batson VD, Yoder LH (2012) Managerial coaching: a concept analysis. J Adv Nurs 68(7):1658–1669. https://doi.org/10.1111/j.1365-2648.2011.05840.x
5. Furtado LC, Batista Mda G, Silva FJ (2011) Leadership and job satisfaction among Azorean hospital nurses: an application of the situational leadership model. J Nurs Manag 19(8):1047–1057. https://doi.org/10.1111/j.1365-2834.2011.01281.x
6. Snow F (2019) Creativity and innovation: an essential competency for the nurse leader. Nurs Adm Q 43(4):306–312. https://doi.org/10.1097/NAQ.0000000000000367
7. Manz CC (1992) Self-leading work teams: moving beyond self-management myths. Human Relat 45(11):1119–1140. https://doi.org/10.1177/001872679204501101
8. The Future of Jobs Report 2020. World Economic Forum. 2020. Available at https://www3.weforum.org/docs/WEF_Future_of_Jobs_2020.pdf
9. Knotts K, Houghton JD, Pearce CL, Chen H, Stewart GL, Manz CC (2022) Leading from the inside out: a meta-analysis of how, when, and why self-leadership affects individual outcomes. Eur J Work and Organizational Psychol 31(2):273–291. https://doi.org/10.1080/1359432X.2021.1953988
10. Ahmed H, Abd Elhamed S (2021) Future foresight: effect of VUCA leadership educational program on nurse manager's readiness for change. ASNJ 9(27):11–20. https://doi.org/10.21608/asnj.2021.102524.1252
11. Bennett N, Lemoine J (2014) What a difference a word makes: understanding threats to performance in a VUCA world. In: Business Horizons. https://doi.org/10.2139/ssrn.2406676. https://ssrn.com/abstract=2406676
12. Akkaya B, Panait M, Apostu SA, Kaya Y (2022) Agile leadership and perceived career success: the mediating role of job embeddedness. Int J Environ Res Public Health 19(8):4834. https://doi.org/10.3390/ijerph19084834
13. Uronen L, Moen H, Teperi S, Martimo KP, Hartiala J, Salanterä S (2020) Towards automated detection of psychosocial risk factors with text mining. Occup Med (Lond) 70(3):203–206. https://doi.org/10.1093/occmed/kqaa022
14. Remegio W, Rivera RR, Griffin MQ, Fitzpatrick JJ (2021) The professional quality of life and work engagement of nurse leaders. Nurse Lead 19(1):95–100. https://doi.org/10.1016/j.mnl.2020.08.001
15. Siirala E, Suhonen H, Salanterä S, Junttila K (2019) The nurse manager's role in perioperative settings: an integrative literature review. J Nurs Manag 27(5):918–929. https://doi.org/10.1111/jonm.12770
16. Siirala E, Peltonen LM, Lundgrén-Laine H, Salanterä S, Junttila K (2016) Nurse managers' decision-making in daily unit operation in peri-operative settings: a cross-sectional descriptive study. J Nurs Manag 27(5):918–929. https://doi.org/10.1111/jonm.12770
17. Cousins B (2018) Design thinking: organizational learning in VUCA environments. ASMJ 17(2):1–18
18. Roberts J, Fisher T, Trowbridge M, Bent C (2016) A design thinking framework for healthcare management and innovation. Healthc (Amst) 4(1):11–14. https://doi.org/10.1016/j.hjdsi.2015.12.002
19. Altman M, Huang TT, Breland JY (2018) Design thinking in health care. Prev Chronic Dis 27(15):E117. https://doi.org/10.5888/pcd15.180128
20. Liedtka J (2018) Why design thinking works. Harv Business Rev 96:72–79
21. Abookire S, Plover C, Frasso R, Ku B (2020) Health design thinking: an innovative approach in public health to defining problems and finding solutions. Front Public Health 28(8):459. https://doi.org/10.3389/fpubh.2020.00459
22. Mortier AV, Vlerick P, Clays E (2016) Authentic leadership and thriving among nurses: the mediating role of empathy. J Nurs Manag 24(3):357–365. https://doi.org/10.1111/jonm.12329
23. Horney N, Pasmore B, O'Shea T (2010) Leadership agility: a business imperative for a VUCA world. People Strategy 33(4):34–42

24. Eines TF, Vatne S (2018) Nurses and nurse assistants' experiences with using a design thinking approach to innovation in a nursing home. J Nurs Manag 26(4):425–431. https://doi.org/10.1111/jonm.12559
25. Tuominen, O. 2022 Rescheduling sudden absences of nursing staff in hospital settings. Turku: University of Turku, Serie D, Medica – Odontologica; 2020; Available from https://www.utupub.fi/handle/10024/148953
26. van Schingen E, Dariel O, Lefebvre H, Challier MP, Rothan-Tondeur M (2017) Mandatory internal mobility in French hospitals: the results of imposed management practices. J Nurs Manag 25(1):4–12. https://doi.org/10.1111/jonm.12417
27. Tuominen O, Lundgren-Laine H, Teperi S, Salanterä S (2020) Comparing the two techniques for nursing staff rescheduling to streamline nurse managers' daily work in Finland. CIN 38(3):148–156. https://doi.org/10.1097/CIN.0000000000000567
28. Hoffman A, von Sadovszky V (2018) Staff nurses' perspectives of resources needed during floating. J Nurs Adm 48(11):580–584. https://doi.org/10.1097/NNA.0000000000000683
29. Lieberman H, Paternò F, Klann M, Wulf V (2006) End-user development: an emerging paradigm. In: Lieberman H, Paternò F, Wulf V (eds) End User Development. Human-Computer Interaction Series, vol 9. Springer, Dordrecht. https://doi.org/10.1007/1-4020-5386-X_1
30. Tuominen OA, Rantalainen T, Löyttyniemi E, Rehnbäck K, Lundgrén-Laine H, Salanterä S (2022) Investigation of the causes and effects of stress in nurses working 'floating shifts'. Nurs Manag (Harrow) 16. https://doi.org/10.7748/nm.2022.e2044

Co-creation and Change in Healthcare

7

Laura Niemi

7.1 Service Ecosystem in Healthcare

Service ecosystems in healthcare consist of multiple actors, networks, and institutional arrangements with such common principles intersecting and overlapping among the micro, meso, and macro levels of social interactions.

Typically, service ecosystems consist of relatively autonomous units operating together with common principles. In general, service ecosystems are dynamic in nature, meaning that each network or actor within the ecosystem can change the nature of the system through resource integration. Within the service ecosystem, different institutions influence the co-creation of value and emphasize the importance of interaction and the social context of the service system as they integrate and recombine resources. Integrating existing resources in a new way by developing new relationships, new services, new processes, and new ways of co-creating value enhances innovations and an emergence of new practices [1, 2].

As described and illustrated above (Fig. 7.1), by definition, the service ecosystem consists of actor networks zooming out from the dyadic relationships while integrating resources from many sources, not only from the service provider or the service user, and these networks are linked by dynamic processes [3]. Although it may be relatively easy to identify the actors and networks involved in a service design process, the systemic thinking about the service ecosystem is often challenging, especially in the context of healthcare service design process which often is implemented by actors that have very different operating cultures [4].

Especially, service providers in the healthcare context mostly perceive service systems differently than the service users do. Hence, healthcare systems are

L. Niemi (✉)
Research Development and Administration, University of Turku, Turku, Finland
e-mail: laura.niemi@utu.fi

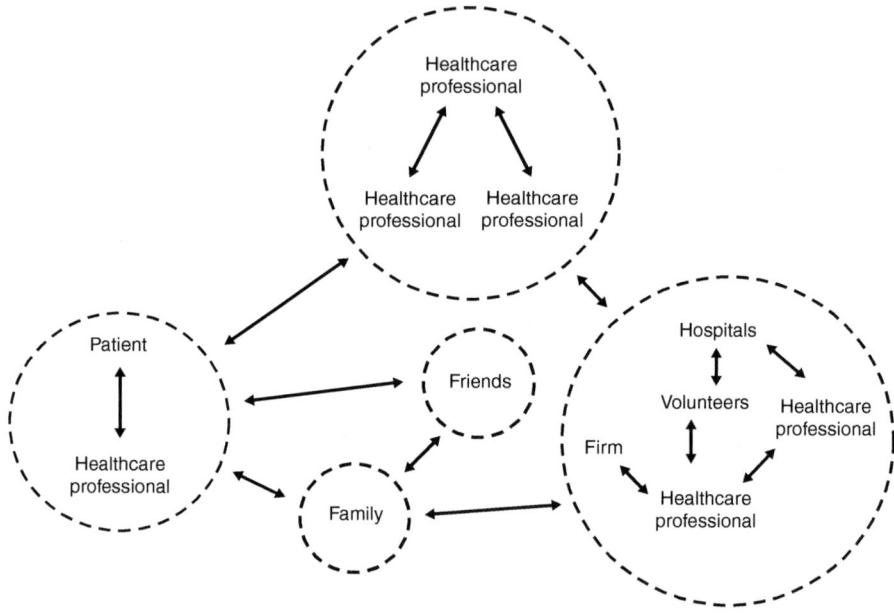

Fig. 7.1 Relationships in service ecosystem (exemplary actor networks)

traditionally planned with organizational considerations in mind, but the resulting systems can appear complex and confusing to the users of the service. For example, users are often forced to navigate a landscape of many separate, uncoordinated services to get the care they need. In some cases, the healthcare systems tend to insufficiently meet the needs of people with rare or complex health or life situations, who may have to use many disparate services offered by several providers such as health centers, hospitals, rehabilitation providers, home care, pharmacies, and social care. Healthcare service providers are often narrowly focused on the treatment of a well-being or the specific illness and, therefore, can fail to consider the overall view of a service user. In health service research, analyzing service in terms of interacting systems of actors and applying the idea of the service design process that extends to whole ecosystem have served as a way to solve such problems (see, e.g. Rossi and Tuurnas [5]).

7.2   Co-creation of Value in Healthcare

Traditionally, healthcare sector has regarded healthcare services as the processes through which people passively receive care from service providers, including, for example, clinicians, nurses, and allied healthcare professionals. Currently, however, the relationship between citizens and healthcare sector has evolved and citizens are increasingly seen as active people who contribute to their health, and therefore, the creation and design of healthcare offerings can no longer emphasize and focus on the delivery of the solutions to passive receivers [6].

This change is reflected in how many healthcare service providers have started to refer to patients as consumers of health. Moreover, the introduction of terminology such as patient engagement [7] and patient-centered care [8] in health service literature is indicating that the role of the service providers is chancing in healthcare.

Despite this change, the healthcare sector and health service literature still largely approach the value as an outcome of certain action which is most often measured in terms of money. This kind of outcome-centered view upholds the idea of a *"goods-dominant logic"* (see e.g. Vargo and Lusch [9]) in which the healthcare service providers are creating services that have intrinsic value for them, and people are solely buying customers who use the offered services. Thus, prevailing understanding about health services largely perpetuates economic and transactional views on value creation.

Recently, however, perspectives on interactivity have begun to replace unidirectional notions of value creation. The discussion has been moving away from linear value creation perspectives toward the existence of more complex and dynamic interaction systems of actors. These perspectives are related to *service-dominant logic* (SD logic) (see, e.g. Vargo and Lusch [9, 10]), which highlights that value is not embedded in produced service outputs and cannot be measured sufficiently in monetary terms.

It is clear that SD logic and service design (i.e. design thinking and patient-centeredness) go hand-in-hand as according to SD logic, value is co-created by multiple actors through interactions in an effort to advance the interests of all actors and the whole system. The essence of SD logic is that value does not arise from internal organization or individual actions. Rather, value arises through the interactions of actors, either directly or through service, in a particular context. Value is co-created reciprocally in interactions among several actors, and new value emerges when resources from various sources are combined in the context of each actor's life [9, 10].

The co-creation of value has led to the understanding that the value emerges in social interactions between people and does not depend on a single person, a single insight, or a single act but on on-going, iterative, and continuous interactions extending well beyond dyadic transactions [3]. This idea of the co-creation of value is quite applicable to the healthcare sector, which forms a complex service ecosystem with multiple internal and external network actors and systems and in which strong motivation exists for creating good and seeking beneficial solutions for the people who are the targets of services.

Although the basic idea of the co-creation of value fits well in healthcare sector, incorporating it into the healthcare service design process is challenging as the healthcare sector is still very often focusing on medical expertise, internal processes, and professional autonomy in decision-making rather than on genuinely collaborating with the multi-professional teams or patients. Yet, from a subjective wellbeing perspective or in complex health conditions, the co-creation of value is broader function than the treatment of a single condition. Hence, in the co-creation the value is the result as well as the goal of an interaction and it can be considered as an exchange among the actors involved in specific interaction

[3]. This makes the interactions an important factor in the design of healthcare services because the interactions comprise comprehensive activities relating to service user experiences. Furthermore, the activities of service design are effective tools that utilize the service user experiences generated via communication and interaction to accomplish the co-creation of value. When service users engage in an interaction during the healthcare service process, they can exchange information or ideas with medical staff, providing a new perspective on the situation and thus generating innovative ways to improve the quality of healthcare service [5, 11].

7.3   Role of the Healthcare User in the Co-creation

Currently in healthcare sector and in health service literature, various perspectives and practices are emerging that define the role of the healthcare user (also referred as customer or patient) in the ecosystem, ranging from seeing the service user as a passive recipient of expert medical care to self-managed care where the service user is seen as an active partner in care and service design processes [4].

Accordingly, in healthcare sector the understanding of ecosystems varies across different organizations and within in them it is possible to distinguish three different perspectives to creation of value: either as a system seen from the service provider's viewpoint (a provider-focused ecosystem), a system based on a shared and collective viewpoint (a distributed ecosystem), or a system anchored in a focal user's viewpoint (a user-focused ecosystem). Thus, it is important to note that these three perspectives do not exclude or supplant each other but rather offer complementary starting points for designing service [12].

7.3.1   The Service Provider-Focused Perspective

The provider-focused perspective is a traditional approach to the creation of value and within it, the actual service has been understood in terms of interactions between actors who directly take part in the service process [13]. In practice, many organizations still view the creation of value in this way as they are taking 'a supply-side' approach to the creation of value and largely ignoring 'a demand-side' of the equation.

However, this perspective is not as narrow as before as the understanding of the actors involved in the creation of value in the service process has extended over time from simple provider-user dyads to more complex service systems. Hence, these service systems are understood as the systems of structures and processes that exist within a service organization. Consequently, the view of service systems upholds a strong intra-organizational focus, mostly concerned with how organizations should manage service processes for service quality. Thus, this perspective entails understanding systems from the provider's viewpoint, focusing on elements and actors within the provider's control (e.g. Grönroos [14]; Lim and Tang [15]).

7.3.2   The Distributed Ecosystem Perspective

The distributed ecosystem perspective has been greatly influenced by the development of SD logic, a flourishing school of thought within marketing and consumer research, that has developed the traditional conceptualization of service further by defining service as systems where all involved actors are to be viewed on equal terms. Consequently, people might be served by not only one service provider but also a whole ecosystem of providers that interact and collaborate to co-create the service provided to the people. A service ecosystem is defined as a *"relatively self-contained, self-adjusting system of resource-integrating actors connected by shared institutional arrangements and mutual value creation through service exchange"* [16].

Thus, the focus is on mutuality and shared institutional arrangements, emphasizing a system that enables a service provision through service-for-service exchange. In healthcare context, similar ideas have earlier been presented in terms of integrated healthcare networks and systems and later in terms of healthcare ecosystems. A person might, for example, need to use several service providers for knee surgery and related physiotherapy or rehabilitation. Thus, the hospital providing the initial surgery and the private physiotherapist supporting the rehabilitation can coordinate as a system for the benefit of the person using the service [10, 16, 17].

The development of SD logic has also changed the role of the service user. Within the classic delivery-focused approach to service, the role of the user (or customer) was mainly to receive and consume the service. Nowadays, however, service providers are increasingly started to view service as a process of co-creation between the provider and user. In this way, all the actors in a service system can, in fact, be understood as actors who are participating into a co-creation of value, rather than simply delivering or consuming a service [6, 18]. Thus, the healthcare user can be seen as being involved in a process of interaction and co-creation with a network of other actors: not just receiving healthcare but also actively contributing to it. In this perspective, value is understood as a system-level construct, co-created by several actors. In practice, on the micro level, the nexus of a distributed ecosystem is on a set of focal relationships, such as physician–patient, patient–healthcare team, or patient–family member (e.g. parent/spouse/sibling/friend), whereas on the meso and macro levels, the nexus is on the links between different types of health and other organizations. Thus, the main objective of managing a service ecosystem is to facilitate mutual value creation and service-to-service exchange [4].

7.3.3   The Service User-Focused Perspective

The service user-focused perspective highlights that people use service beyond the control of individual service providers. Thus, in the service user sphere, the service provider has limited influence and the user is actually more in control of the service design process, acting according to their own goals, motives, and life themes [19].

This perspective takes its starting point in the user's processes and the user's own subjective understanding of what is valuable and helpful for the individual person who uses the service. Thus, the user's goals for engaging with a set of actors and services that form an ecosystem are to enable wellbeing for themselves and for other relevant parties. The actual service ecosystem then consists of services, actors, elements, and technologies that are identified from the point of view of the user's own value-creating process. Hence, this perspective views service and value from the user's individual and idiosyncratic viewpoint [20, 21].

Crucially, users' value-creating processes often go beyond the scope of touch-points and interactions in planned service processes. This implies that individual service users join directly and indirectly together as dyads, triads, and complex. These active individuals are also involved in a multitude of co-existing interactions and build situational relations with their social surroundings by interacting with others through practices, rituals, or traditions to create relationships among and identities for themselves [12, 19, 22].

Thus, the service users are creating an environment that in the end becomes a social system of individuals in which the recourses are integrated, the new services are accepted, and, ultimately, new value is defined and co-created with service providers but also independently from interactions with the service providers. Accordingly, the actual value of the service is determined not only by individual perceptions of value-in-use but also by wider social perceptions. Therefore, the value of the service should be understood as *"value-in-social-context"* [23], because an individual's perceptions and experiences of new value depend, at least to some extent, on the individual's relative position within the wider social context.

7.4   Toward an Interaction-Based Approach to Healthcare Service

Healthcare sector can be characterized as a service ecosystem of multiple actors in which the creation of value has shifted from being a top-down process of a single service provider to an interactive process of many actors. Thus, co-creation opens the healthcare service designing and development up to a wide range of voices that would normally never be involved.

The systemic thinking combined with the understanding of the user-focused perspective promotes an interaction-based approach to healthcare service design process. A well-designed healthcare service process should recognize that people are not objects of a treatment or some other activity but active co-producers of the service who are actively involved in the co-creation of value.

From a service provider perspective, there are two factors that have a particular impact on the service provider's service design process:

1. the user entity and
2. the value-creating activities

The first factor that impacts the service design process is the user entity. The user entity could be, for example, a family or another group of people acting collectively. Thus, a user entity can be a unified group of people who share goals and directly influence each other in terms of service use, choices, and support. For example, a couple, where one has fallen seriously ill, can form a user unit. Both people are involved in treating the disease and are affected by its events and outcomes. The person who has fallen sick sets the initial scope of the service provider by means of their insurance and public and private service providers, for example, while the spouse may bring in additional actors and elements in terms of discussions with associations and peer group activities, as well as family and friends, and so on. Thus, the assembly of people in the user entity defines the scope of the actual service ecosystem. Therefore, a successful service design process requires decisions to be made on the user entity at the center of the service ecosystem.

The second factor, the value-creating activities, refers to what the user entity collectively wants to achieve or do. In healthcare, this could be considered narrowly as the actors or services involved in a linear process to treat a specific disease or condition or, from a wider perspective, as the actors involved a set of everyday events that relate to maintaining or improving a person's health on a more general level. The value-creating activities of an ecosystem can be defined according to the user entity's ultimate goal. Depending on which goal is chosen, a specific set of actors or services will be highlighted and others are excluded. Further, this means that a single user entity may maintain many overlapping ecosystems that relate to different, interrelated user goals. For example, there may be one ecosystem that supports everyday mental health, another supporting general wellbeing, and a third for treating a particular disease. These ecosystems are partly overlapping, and all contribute to the general subjective wellbeing of the user entity. Thus, the service user may have multi-touch points and multi-channel (e.g. devices, applications, and face-to-face exchange) encounters in their service journey; the co-creation of value can occur through a variety of interactions. Therefore, it is important for the healthcare service provider to consider how different user experiences can be maximized through a healthcare service design process [3].

7.5 Co-creation as Enabler of Reform and Change in Healthcare Service

The objective of this chapter is to increase understanding of value co-creation of the services. The ultimate goal is to approach issues from a new perspective that makes it possible to achieve better healthcare services, products, and processes. Since the premise of the co-creation of value is that several actors contribute to a collective effort in co-creation, the resulting service, product, or process is theoretically valuable for all actors involved.

Recently the health service literature has focused on value co-creation in healthcare services and the importance of engaging patients and other actors in service delivery, and patient participation in the co-creation of value has been shown to improve expected service outcomes. Thus, the increased interaction within the healthcare service design process between service users and service provider is a critical factor for improving care quality and user satisfaction. This is especially evident when service users must frequently engage in interactions with the service provider. Thus, at the beginning of the service design process, the healthcare service provider should examine how all actors within the recognized service ecosystem can interact with service users at various encounters, and how different actors and organizations can provide needed facilities or information to create effective touchpoints, such as medical facilities, websites, devices, and applications, that are valuable for service users and enhance the effective use of the healthcare service.

Moreover, the change and transformation of healthcare services and the creation of new healthcare services call for collaboration within the service ecosystem to carefully define the new service design processes and new roles in that process. Thus, this requires high managerial involvement in ensuring that new service design processes can be integrated into the working processes of an organization.

The healthcare ecosystem consists of systems and professionals in various areas of medicine, nursing, therapy, IT, and law, among others. In responding to the challenge digitization sets for the services, the expertise of all actors is needed in order to establish complete and consistent services that also meet the requirements for medical devices set by regulations and legislative norms (e.g. European Committee [24]). The actor network integrates these resources and relevant information in the development of the system, as well as in defining the practices for care or treatment through the service.

The new approach outlined in this chapter can help healthcare professionals and service providers understand the role of the services they are trying to control, in relation to other relevant, hidden services and actors within the service ecosystem in which they operate. However, before any change or new service can be created, the service providers need to understand the relevant user unit, which also might be hidden from an external actor's perspective. Only after recognizing the user unit, it is possible to start uncovering the other steps in the service design process. This allows the leaders of the healthcare service design process to discover how their preconceived notions of an ecosystem may differ from the actual service ecosystem. By understanding the role and position of their service from the user-focused perspective, the leaders in the healthcare service design process may better be able to support their users' everyday value-creating processes.

Moreover, a service provider may have different roles in different, parallel healthcare service processes, depending on what value-creating function it supports. By understanding the service from the user-focused perspective, service provider can also discover which other actors they might need to collaborate or communicate with. Notably, the healthcare professionals and the leaders in the healthcare service design process can use insights about individual user ecosystems in planning patient-centered care.

References

1. Vargo SL, Wieland H, Akaka MA (2015) Innovation through institutionalization: a service ecosystems perspective. Ind Mark Manag [Internet] 44:63–72. Available from:. https://doi.org/10.1016/j.indmarman.2014.10.008
2. Akaka MA, Vargo SL (2015) Extending the context of service: from encounters to ecosystems. J Serv Mark [Internet] 29(6/7):453–462. Available from:. https://doi.org/10.1108/jsm-03-2015-0126
3. Brodie RJ, Fehrer JA, Jaakkola E, Conduit J (2019) Actor engagement in networks: Defining the conceptual domain. J Serv Res [Internet] 22(2):173–188. Available from:. https://doi.org/10.1177/1094670519827385

4. McColl-Kennedy JR, Cheung L, Coote LV (2020) Tensions and trade-offs in multi-actor service ecosystems. J Bus Res [Internet]. 121:655–666. Available from:. https://doi.org/10.1016/j.jbusres.2020.06.055

5. Rossi P, Tuurnas S (2021) Conflicts fostering understanding of value co-creation and service systems transformation in complex public service systems. Publ Manag Rev [Internet] 23(2):254–275. Available from:. https://doi.org/10.1080/14719037.2019.1679231

6. McColl-Kennedy JR, Hogan SJ, Witell L, Snyder H (2017) Cocreative customer practices: effects of health care customer value cocreation practices on well-being. J Bus Res [Internet] 70:55–66. Available from:. https://doi.org/10.1016/j.jbusres.2016.07.006

7. Barello S, Graffigna G, Vegni E (2012) Patient engagement as an emerging challenge for healthcare services: mapping the literature. Nurs Res Pract 2012:905934. Available from. https://doi.org/10.1155/2012/905934

8. Epstein RM, Street RL Jr (2011) The values and value of patient-centered care. Ann Fam Med 9(2):100–103. Available from:. https://doi.org/10.1370/afm.1239

9. Vargo SL, Lusch RF (2004) Evolving to a new dominant logic for marketing. J Mark 68(1):1–17. Available from:. https://doi.org/10.1509/jmkg.68.1.1.24036

10. Vargo SL, Lusch RF (2017) Service-dominant logic 2025. Int J Res Mark 34(1):46–67. Available from:. https://doi.org/10.1016/j.ijresmar.2016.11.001

11. Hardyman W, Kitchener M, Daunt KL (2019) What matters to me! User conceptions of value in specialist cancer care. Publ Manag Rev 21(11):1687–1706. Available from:. https://doi.org/10.1080/14719037.2019.1619808

12. Mickelsson J, Särkikangas U, Strandvik T, Heinonen K (2022) User-defined ecosystems in health and social care. J Serv Mark 36(9):41–56. Available from:. https://doi.org/10.1108/jsm-03-2021-0090

13. Parasuraman A, Zeithaml VA, Berry LL (1985) A conceptual model of service quality and its implications for future research. J Mark 49(4):41–50. Available from:. https://doi.org/10.1177/002224298504900403

14. Grönroos C (2000) Service management and marketing: a customer relationship management approach. John Wiley and Sons, Ltd.

15. Cheng Lim P, Tang NKH (2000) The development of a model for total quality healthcare. Manag Serv Qual 10(2):103–111. Available from:. https://doi.org/10.1108/09604520010318290

16. Vargo SL, Lusch RF (2016) Institutions and axioms: an extension and update of service-dominant logic. J Acad Mark Sci 44(1):5–23. Available from: doi:10.1007/s11747-015-0456-3 15

17. Frow P, McColl-Kennedy JR, Payne A, Govind R (2019) Service ecosystem well-being: conceptualization and implications for theory and practice. Eur J Mark 53(12):2657–2691. Available from:. https://doi.org/10.1108/ejm-07-2018-0465

18. Frow P, McColl-Kennedy JR, Payne A (2016) Co-creation practices: their role in shaping a health care ecosystem. Ind Mark Manag 56:24–39. Available from:. https://doi.org/10.1016/j.indmarman.2016.03.007

19. Heinonen K, Strandvik T, Mickelsson K-J, Edvardsson B, Sundström E, Andersson P (2010) A customer-dominant logic of service. J Serv Manag 21(4):531–548. Available from:. https://doi.org/10.1108/09564231011066088

20. Heinonen K, Strandvik T, Voima P (2013) Customer dominant value formation in service. Eur Bus Rev 25(2):104–123. Available from:. https://doi.org/10.1108/09555341311302639

21. Heinonen K, Strandvik T (2020) Customer-dominant service logic. In: The Routledge Handbook of Service Research Insights and Ideas. Routledge, New York, pp 69–89

22. Grönroos C, Voima P (2013) Critical service logic: making sense of value creation and co-creation. J Acad Mark Sci 41(2):133–150. Available from:. https://doi.org/10.1007/s11747-012-0308-3

23. Edvardsson B, Tronvoll B, Gruber T (2011) Expanding understanding of service exchange and value co-creation: a social construction approach. J Acad Mark Sci 39(2):327–339. Available from:. https://doi.org/10.1007/s11747-010-0200-y

24. European Committee (2007) Health informatics: system of concepts to support continuity of care. Part 1: Basic concepts. European Committee for Standardization, Brussels, Belgium

New Business Creation in Health Technology

8

Kaapo Seppälä

8.1 Medical Devices and Regulatory Environment

The health technology sector is highly regulated, and internationally the legal and regulatory requirements for medical devices are very complex. To place a product classified as a medical device on the EU market, a company must comply with the legislation in force at every stage of product development. The CE mark appears on the product as a sign of compliance with regulatory requirements. The regulation is not limited to the product development phase, but covers all aspects of the company's activities and products throughout their life cycle. The responsibility of the company starts at the product development stage and continues even after the products have been placed on the market. In practice, companies use international standards to develop a compliant product. For the CE mark, the most relevant are the EU harmonized standards. There are around 300 of these harmonized standards used in the health technology sector and some of the most important include:

- ISO 13485 Medical devices—Quality management systems—Requirements for regulatory purposes
- ISO 14971 Medical devices—Application of risk management to medical devices
- EN 62304 Medical device software—Software lifecycle processes.

Other standards used were the risk management standard ISO 14971, the usability standard IEC 62366, and the software development lifecycle model IEC 62304.

K. Seppälä (✉)
Faculty of Technology, University of Turku, Turku, Finland
e-mail: kaapo.seppala@utu.fi

101

For example, the manufacturer must use standards to show that the product meets the essential requirements based on legislation. In practice, it is very difficult to demonstrate compliance with the law unless you rely on standards. A new version of the quality management standard ISO 13485 was published on 1 March 2016. This new version of the standard brought changes to which the industry has had to react. During the time of the survey, the standard became a top priority issue for most of the companies in medical device sector also in Finland.

So how the relevant companies reacted? Three different groups of companies emerged from the interview material in terms of quality management. The first group consists of companies that comply with ISO 13485 because their product is clearly a medical device or they feel that compliance with the standard is a status issue and brings credibility to the product and the company. The second group is made up of companies that do not comply with ISO1385 because their product does not require it and they feel it is too expensive and complex for their needs. The third group consists of companies that wonder whether compliance with ISO 13485 would give them a competitive advantage and allow them to participate in more competitions [1].

The interviews clearly showed the importance of the regulatory aspect. Companies that did not find regulations and regulatory requirements problematic said that they did so because they had skilled staff with experience in areas such as product approvals or quality management. Conversely, companies without staff with experience in a regulatory background reported that it was difficult to free up resources to set up a quality management system, for example, when it was needed for product development or sales, for example. Companies had plans to hire a person or persons to deal with regulatory requirements as their business grew. Some companies had hired a part-time person to deal with quality management issues, and the use of consultants was also common among respondents. Recruitment and training of in-house staff were used to acquire expertise.

Regulatory expertise was also seen as a competitive advantage. For example, during the time of the interviews, Estonia was not considered a significant competitor to Finland in the health technology sector due to its demanding approval procedures and quality management. Decisions to keep production in Finland are also often based on the fact that quality is easier to control when production takes place nearby [1].

In summary, regulatory requirements and quality management were seen by some companies as an isolated stage, rather than as an essential part of product development. The high level of use of consultants reflects in part the complexity of the issue and the fact that small and new companies in particular do not have the necessary skills and resources to deal with regulatory issues. However, extensive use of consultants does not necessarily build up the skills of the company. It can also be a challenge to find and select competent consultants if the company does not have the experience and contacts in place. On the other hand, the stringent requirements for product development of medical devices give a competitive advantage to companies that master them.

8.2   Defining the Customer

As a starting point, the customer and the customer's needs are as essential in the health technology sector as in any other. However, defining the customer and the user is a complex issue. Ultimately, the customer is the patient and their health, both from a preventive and health problem-solving perspective. Therefore, the starting point for the development of a healthcare device must be an understanding of the medical context, for example, for the diagnosis or treatment of the patient [1]. The patient, especially for lower-risk devices, is also the actual user of the device. However, the user is often a healthcare professional, for example, a doctor or nurse, who is then the more relevant decision maker for the purchase decision, even if the product will ultimately be used for the benefit of the patient. Purchasing behavior varies from country to country, and there are also major differences between public health services and private health service providers. Particularly on the public side, the purchaser may be a purchasing professional, which sometimes brings its own challenges in ensuring that the purchase decision is based on the suitability of the device to solve a medical problem and not just on price. Once a device is on the market, the success of the sale, especially if it is a very new approach, also depends on its cost-benefit acceptability to society. This issue is addressed by Health Technology Assessment analyses and it may influence Current Care recommendations.

Product innovation alone is not enough. Ultimately, the starting point for the development of a healthcare device must be the patient's needs and the user's needs, for example, to diagnose or treat a patient. Therefore, understanding the medical problem and the needs of the patient and the user must be thoroughly investigated in the early stages of product development. A product that delivers real health benefits and quantified added value over competitors has greater probability to be successful.

The customer and customer needs are equally relevant to regulatory requirements. Based on these, the manufacturer defines the intended use of the product, which determines whether the product is a healthcare device or not. It also influences the risk classification of the product. As an official requirement, the characteristics of the final product must be aligned with the product specifications of the product development baseline, which in turn must be based on user needs [1].

8.3   Entering the Markets

In many cases, health-related research carried out at universities has laid the foundations for the emergence of health technology businesses, although researchers themselves are still relatively rarely entrepreneurs themselves. Business opportunities may also have arisen as large players have concentrated their business activities, for example, by downsizing or offshoring.

In companies, the support of national public R&D funding (Business Finland, Vinnova, etc.) has often played an important role in the product development phase.

Incubators and mentoring programs such as Spark Finland or universities' own commercialization programs have also helped the sector to enter the market. For example, an incubator may have provided a company with a budget for preparing commercialization, for example, to carry out market research and identify funding opportunities. This may have enabled companies to secure their first contracts for the distribution of their products.

Companies often develop their products from an innovative and technological point of view. However, the conditions for success exist only if there is a good understanding of international markets, customers, customer needs, and buying behavior. From Finnish perspective, health technology products are mostly aimed at international markets. One-third of products remain in the EU, one-third in the US, and the remaining third in other parts of the world. In order to export, a company needs to know the international market and create a marketing strategy in the early stages of product development. Depending on the countries targeted, the customers and their needs may be very different. Different countries will also face different regulatory requirements and their impact on product specifications, how the product is developed, produced, and ultimately marketed can be very different. Without a marketing strategy, one cannot develop a sound regulatory strategy and without it, one cannot develop a product that meets the regulatory requirements of the chosen target country. A medical device must comply with regulatory requirements and the company is also subject to requirements for quality management systems. For example, only compliant devices can be CE marked in the EU, and a device without a CE mark is not allowed to be placed on the market.

8.4   Sales

SMEs see the health sector as rather conservative. Bringing new solutions to the sector is seen to be requiring quite a lot of influencing of authorities. In terms of sales, it is important that the company try to create a credible enough image for itself, for example, through scientific publishing and communication. In Finland, for example, it is felt that Finnish healthcare customers are inclined to buy products from leading American manufacturers in particular, as most are familiar with these manufacturers and their resources, visibility, and influence are so great [1]. Small firms can try to compete against large foreign players by knowing customers personally, being close to them and thus trying to serve them as well as possible.

Most companies actively participate in industry fairs and events. Trade fairs provide an opportunity, among other things, to get feedback, to find out where operators are interested, and to make contacts for R&D project applications. This information can be used to identify where to take the company's product, how to better target its marketing, and how to find partners in the future. Entrepreneurs see that you need to market your product in this way for a few years and meet customers in person at events a few times before you can actually start selling to them [1].

In terms of their target market, very few health technology companies have focused exclusively on the consumer market. The majority of companies had the largest number of institutional customers, with the largest number of sales to public sector customers. Of the Finnish respondents to the 2017 survey, about half sold mainly to the public sector, about a quarter sold mainly to the private sector, and about a quarter sold roughly equally to both target groups [1]. Regarding regulatory requirements, it should be noted that requirements in the consumer market are much more stringent than if the device is sold to a healthcare professional.

As the majority of products are very often sold outside the national borders and often also outside the EU, manufacturers rarely have the opportunity to sell their products themselves. At the outset, the size of the company may not allow it to set up its own subsidiaries, sales organizations, except perhaps in the most important markets. In such cases, the creation of an effective network of distributors remains a more viable option. It is worth starting to build up sales channels early enough, as the process of finding, evaluating, contracting, and training a distributor can easily take months, even years. Whatever the sector, sufficient effort must be invested in contracts, using international expertise—different countries may be affected by very different legislation. In health technology contracts or their annexes, it must be remembered that specific regulations in the sector must be carefully highlighted. For example, the responsibilities of the manufacturer and distributor in handling complaints, reporting incidents, and recalls should be taken into account. Similarly, the ownership of registrations, the responsibilities of the distributor/importer/authorized representative, and the correctness of marketing materials and practices need to be clearly agreed.

8.5 Thoughts About Business Models

In terms of business model, small start-ups and original equipment manufacturers (OEMs) sell primarily on a one-off basis. This is done because of the need to generate revenue up front and the inability or unwillingness to commit resources to equipment. On the other hand, potential OEM customers may only want the equipment and develop the software or other additional services themselves. In such a situation, the possibilities to offer the product as a service, or even to offer services that complement the solution at all, are reduced. In all cases, the regulatory requirements must be respected and the manufacturer is responsible for the intended use, features, use, and usability of the product.

In any case, selling as a service is seen as a business opportunity. Many companies are considering selling as a service in an effort to move their business in a direction that enables them to do so (e.g., by investing resources in in-house service development). On the other hand, there is a decreasing willingness of customers to invest in equipment and other facilities, which supports the use of a service-based business model.

Ancillary services sold by companies include IQ (installation qualification), OQ (operational qualification), and maintenance services. These services are provided after installation and ensure that the equipment is operational. Depending on the customer, universities, for example, are generally not interested in purchasing qualification services, but customer companies operating under a quality system often are. Healthcare services may well be interested in such ancillary services.

Additional services that companies perceive as most important for their turnover (percentage of companies) [1]:

1. User training 25%
2. Operational support services (advice, guidance) 23%
3. Out-of-warranty after-sales services 16%
4. Product updates 16%
5. Installation services 13%
6. Analysis services 7%

Training and support services are often perceived by companies as the most important services in terms of sales, although they are not usually charged for separately.

When sold as a service, the product is used through a service provider, which means that, at least in principle, companies are also well placed to provide value-added services related to the data collected by the device in one form or another. This kind of business has increased together with awareness concerning the IoT (Internet of Things) technology. However, in the context of data collection, customers may be in the habit of using certain devices connected to offline computers, as there can be seen a risk that the network connection may interfere with the devices. In some cases, the use of the network connection may also be prohibited. In these cases the device will naturally not be able to provide the company with usage data. Sensitive data collected via devices must also be anonymized when it arrives at the company's servers. The system must therefore be built in such a way that companies do not have access to patient data, which they must also be able to demonstrate to the customer.

Product usage data is more difficult to apply in product development, as the product is already finished when it is used and cannot be changed once it has been approved in a certain form. No product can be delivered to the customer until it is ready and meets all criteria, including regulatory requirements. The product must be 'frozen,' so that it can only be modified in accordance with a specific process.

Some companies have stated that the original equipment manufacturer (OEM) model has been effective in the early stages of a company, when there was no distribution network and no major resources to bring a product to market. The disadvantage of being an OEM supplier is that there is an intermediary between the company and the user of the product, so that user feedback is received through an intermediary and naturally filtered along the way [1].

In order to lower the threshold for purchasing a product, many companies offer to test their product in the customer's environment. For example, in the case of one company selling on a one-off basis, the customer can first have a 3-month trial of the product. The customer pays a few thousand euros, which is credited to the total price if he decides to keep the device. This was seen as facilitating the customer's decision to purchase.

8.6   Main Challenges Facing the Industry

According to the 2017 survey, by far the biggest challenge in the health technology industry was the creation of sales channels, which was ranked by a majority of respondents as one of the top three challenges. The second important challenge was regulation and regulatory requirements. Around a third of the respondents selected 'other problems' as the biggest challenges, including challenges in accessing finance and challenges in growing the business [1].

Other key challenges include also defining/choosing a business model, increasing competition, insufficient demand, decreasing customer willingness/ability to pay, increasing labor costs, and increasing other costs [1].

In addition to the challenges mentioned above, some firms perceive 'market harassment' from some companies, that is, firms that have received large amounts of capital investment, as a problem. For example, if there is a lot of capital available in China at certain point, and if a company receives such a large capital injection, it is very difficult to compete with them.

Main challenges that companies perceive as most relevant for their business (percentage of companies mentioning a certain challenge, $N=32$) [1]:

1. Managing sales channels 81%
2. Regulatory environment 68%
3. Business model 50%
4. Low demand, low willingness to pay 31%
5. Costs increase 28%
6. Competition 19%
7. Recruiting challenges 9%
8. Other reasons 31%

Many of the challenges mentioned above are such that they can be said affecting the whole field of technology sales in general. However, a challenge specific to the health technology sector is the regulation of national healthcare and in particular, the law on tendering.

Changes in legislation and standards are a challenge, as the workforce is not always available to respond to them. This underlines the importance of having the right consultant. In addition, situations where a product is about to be launched on a new market or is being considered for CE marking often require new skills.

In the case of public customers, national tendering laws and practices are seen as a particular challenge, as many respondents felt that they limit the dialogue between the buyer and the suppliers. In addition, in large organizations, the person responsible for tendering may not always be up to date with the latest technology and this can lead to poor criteria for the customer or end-user when selecting a product. Calls for tenders may also include, for example, a requirement for the company's turnover, which may in practice exclude most SMEs from tendering, regardless of their quality and performance.

Competition from Asia is also seen as a challenge, as many operators import competing products from China. European companies themselves regularly order competing products to test them, as customers are also constantly scanning the market.

Long product development cycles require funding, and many European companies often seek to attract venture capital at some stage to secure their own business and competitive position. In some countries, such as Finland, it is felt that the investor culture is not yet sufficiently developed and capital can be difficult to obtain. The long product development cycles of health technology products also require long-term investors who can wait for a return. The Nordic countries welcome the support mechanisms and institutions (e.g., Business Finland, Vinnova) for the product development phase as they invest heavily in financing SMEs. However, the 2017 survey felt that there should be more support opportunities for companies also after the product development phase. The so-called *valley of death* is the stage when the product can be ready, but the company does not yet have the cash flow to cover its costs. Support would be needed at this stage, especially as market entry with limited resources is perceived as challenging in any case.

Challenges in the operating environment include the fact that the quality of products supplied by subcontractors is not always up to standard, causing unnecessary delays in the production chain.

8.7   Implications to the Product Development

One of the key goals of a manufacturing company is to drive product development so that new needs and technologies can be identified and brought to market before competitors. The aim is to reduce development times, lower product development costs, and better satisfy customer needs [2].

In industries such as health technology, knowledge and attention to the regulatory environment in product development, manufacturing, and sales also give a company a significant competitive advantage, as the interview data suggest. Being aware of regulations from the outset speeds up market entry and reduces the number of extra iterations, in this case moving to an earlier stage of development.

User-centered design, in turn, can reduce the time needed for overall product design and possible redesign. User-centered design methods also make it easier to identify and act on problems earlier, thus reducing the cost of change.

A company designing its first health technology device needs to be able to simultaneously document its product development process and discuss its needs with the customer. At the same time, the company must also be able to address the needs of the customer as far as possible by applying user-centered design. The more regulated the industry, the more challenging it becomes to integrate the sales process with this type of product development and regulatory environment (Fig. 8.1).

The first stage of product development, the pre-design phase, involves defining the intended use and identifying requirements. The definition of the intended use determines if the device is a healthcare device in the first place and which category

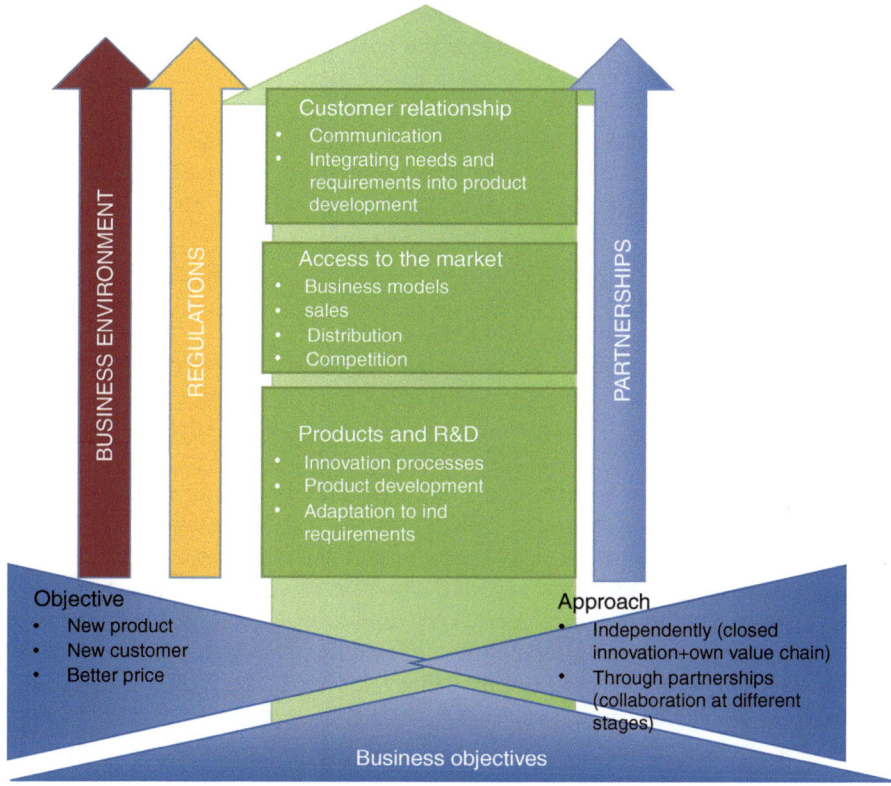

Fig. 8.1 External factors that affect the value chain [1]

of device it belongs to. The purpose of use largely determines the requirements to be met by the device [3]. In practice, this means that, for example, the requirements for a device in a hospital setting are often different from those in a non-clinical setting.

In the case of medical devices, a product class has to be defined, which is divided into classes I, IIa, IIb, and III based on the risk level and on the intended use. The classification is based, inter alia, on (European Parliament [4]):

- duration of use;
- the part of the body with which the equipment comes into contact;
- whether the device is inside the body;
- whether it has its own energy source.

The requirements increase according to the category of product. The definition of the product category is done by the company itself and this definition is one of the essential steps at the beginning of the development process. If the manufacturer is unable to meet the requirements of the product class, a lower product class must be pursued.

Regardless of whether product development is done in-house or with the help of partners, requirements definition reduces the need for additional iterations in the product development process. This saves time and costs. The pre-design phase must also include risk management throughout the process [5].

Product development must also include the production of the necessary documentation (technical documentation for the device, product labeling, and instructions for use, clinical evaluation, declaration of conformity, and device registration) [3].

Selling a device, for example, to a hospital, does not automatically mean that it should be registered as a medical device. Nevertheless, it may be subject to the same safety requirements as healthcare equipment [3, 5].

When considering customer and user needs for the R&D, it should be noted that the customer and the end-user may be the same person, but typically, the person deciding on the purchase of industrial equipment is not the user of the equipment being purchased.

Between the producer and the end-user, there may be several different actors, such as equipment agents, with their own interests. It is important to identify the different actors involved in the procurement process so that product development can take their requirements into account. The role of vendors in managing customer relations is generally considered to be crucial, especially in a sector such as health technology, where start-ups find it difficult to reach institutional customers in particular. However, it should be noted that sales representatives often represent several different devices or manufacturers and that their work is generally focused on existing products rather than on customer contacts at the development stage (Fig. 8.2).

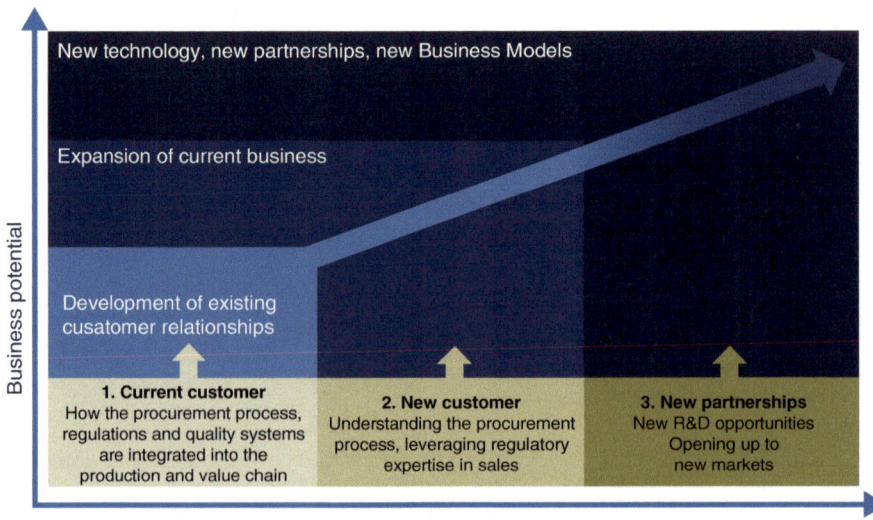

Fig. 8.2 External factors that affect the value chain [1]

In Finland, for example, there is a lot of development work in health technology, and even small companies have a lot of valuable knowledge and industrial property rights as a result. In some cases, however, customer requirements combined with regulations can be so costly for a company that it either has to start developing the product with another company under the same roof (e.g., through a merger) or alternatively sell the whole process to another player (acquisition). Traditionally, mergers are aimed at strengthening market position, market expansion, cost efficiency, synergies, control of product development costs, and dominance in terms of size. In the health technology sector, regulatory constraints or the difficulty of reaching institutional customers may be the starting point for acquisitions or mergers, as otherwise the product cannot be brought to the customer.

References

1. Grönlund M, Ranti T, Raitoharju R, Seppälä K, Ståhlberg T (2017) Suomen terveysteknologia-alan nykytila ja haasteet. Tekes
2. Bruce M, Cooper R (2000) Creative product design. A practical guide for requirements capture management. Wiley, New York
3. Ståhlberg T (2015) Terveydenhuollon laitteiden lakisääteiset määräykset kansainvälisillä markkinoilla Suomi ja EU fokuksessa. Helsinki, Tekes
4. Directive 2007/47/EC of the European Parliament and of the Council of 5 September 2007 amending Council Directive 90/385/EEC on the approximation of the laws of the Member States relating to active implantable medical devices, Council Directive 93/42/EEC concerning medical devices and Directive 98/8/EC concerning the placing of biocidal products on the market.
5. Rane E (2016) The definition and consideration of the requirement specifications of medical devices in company's product development process. Aalto yliopisto

What is the Importance of Design Thinking for Future Healthcare?

Thomas Lemström

9.1 Introduction

This chapter looks beyond the internal workings of design thinking as a methodology. It discusses the importance of design thinking for the future of healthcare and, as such, it requires viewing *the phenomenon of design thinking* from a rather broad perspective. We may even see healthcare going one way with design thinking, and another without it.

This chapter mostly builds upon the author's viewpoint as a practitioner of business design in the field of health innovation. Yet, certain theoretical concepts have survived those practical experiences especially well, and they provide a loose framework for developing the argument presented herein. The key theories influencing the author's thinking are effectuation [1] to explain entrepreneurial action and institutional logics [2] for identifying mechanisms of change and innovation in various socio-cultural contexts.

To answer the question in the title of this chapter, design thinking is discussed, first, in relation to other disciplines typically recognized when discussing innovation. Then it is explained briefly how grassroots-based design thinking is needed to complement and counterbalance the schemes of centralized planning bureaucracies whose reforms tend to fail to create profound change. The third section develops a similar theme wherein the grassroots-based design thinking approach is contrasted to forces of technological imperative and medicalization. Finally, some conclusions are provided regarding how this book and design thinking more generally can be brought to life and why, indeed, design thinking is important for future healthcare.

T. Lemström (✉)
SPARK Finland, Turku, Finland
e-mail: thomas.lemstrom@sparkfinland.fi

© The Author(s), under exclusive license to Springer Nature
Switzerland AG 2023
A. Pakarinen et al. (eds.), *Design Thinking in Healthcare*,
https://doi.org/10.1007/978-3-031-24510-7_9

9.2   Important Vs. Important

Clearly, this book is here to make the case for design thinking, and its importance for the future of healthcare. But how may we characterize its importance? It seems there are at least two ways that the importance of various disciplines is understood. This is elucidated in the following anecdote.

The author attended a meeting where results of a survey were discussed. A group of managers (at universities engaged in medical research and innovation) had been asked to rate the importance of various competencies needed to turn academic discoveries into practical solutions and new businesses. In their responses the number one position was captured by the rather vague term "business development" followed by "finance," "regulation," and "intellectual property management."

Strategy, design, and entrepreneurship were mentioned way down the list. However, it can be argued that they provide far greater potential for widening the bottlenecks of innovation than the topics that had ended up topping the survey. What explains the discrepancy?

The problem might lie in the wording of the survey question. Especially the term "important" can be misleading. It often refers to something that is associated with high social rank, influence, prominence, position, and authority. In the light of these criteria, regulation and intellectual property rights do indeed appear *important*. Moreover, managers in academia, corporations, and healthcare are conditioned to survive within meritocratic hierarchies and administrative bureaucracies. Therefore, they might value the formal, centralized, and established over the informal, decentralized, and explorative. In other words, their answers might reflect an administrative-managerialist bias.

There is another way to understand what "important" means. It can stand for something that strongly affects the course of events or the nature of things. Design thinking, strategic choice, and entrepreneurial capabilities strongly affect the process of innovation. Indeed, they are paramount whereas having sufficient knowledge on finance, regulation, and legal issues are mere *table stakes*. It means that you need them just to have *a seat at the table*, but you need more to *get ahead in the game*, so to speak.

While innovation in healthcare tends to require considerable investments into R&D and compliance with rather complex rules and regulations, these *table stakes* do not provide vision, content, and direction for the innovation process. Those can be facilitated systematically by applying various approaches of design thinking.

9.3   Grassroots and Ivory Towers

In healthcare, as in all complex socio-technical systems, there are grassroots (the *ordinary* work), and there are ivory towers (the *important*, high-status work). Formal schemes like policies, regulations, reform programs, and so on are imposed from the ivory towers of centralized planning bureaucracies upon the unruly grassroots.

Centralized schemes are built on conceptual simplifications of the reality that the grassroots deal with every day [3].

Centralized (top-down) reforms in healthcare have proven problematic, and even quite futile. They are typically driven by vested interests and ideological underpinnings, and they exert influence and requirements on organizations that often steal the space from more pragmatic development efforts. Reforms produce various restructurings that take place within an *administrative paradigm* that survives unaffected by the reforms [4–10].

For instance, administratively driven change has taken place in the Finnish healthcare system over the past few decades mostly through incremental layering of service requirements, structures, and regulations [7, 11, 12]. Innovative changes have been arduous to achieve despite of significant funding [13]. In the end there has been a lot of *reform*, but very little meaningful change.

The tension between grassroots and ivory towers is a part of the context where design thinking takes place. The defense of ideological positions and vested interests forms hurdles to the emergence and adoption of innovations. Innovators and change-makers in healthcare need to be aware of such issues, while those should not be allowed to fan the flames of frustration or cynicism. It merely means that driving change needs to be strategic, and it needs recognition of existing structures, interests, and habitual ways of thinking.

The functioning and renewal of complex socio-technical systems are much more reliant on informal and tacit knowledge that often gets recognized. When push comes to shove, grassroots efforts maintain the whole system via "the indispensable role of practical knowledge, informal processes, and improvisation in the face of unpredictability" [3]. Practical knowledge, familiarity of informal processes, and ability to improvise are raw material for creative solutions if they are allowed to flourish. By being human-centric and promoting empathy, design thinking gives voice to grassroots experiences and empowers individuals. Thereby, it creates fertile ground for innovative ideas and experimentation.

While innovations shape the world, they are reciprocally shaped by prevailing structures. As innovation matures and becomes more widely accepted, it also becomes more congruent with established structures and practices. Informal *fringe* ideas and general ideals evolve into more formalized mechanisms of control. Inexplicit ideas are developed and structured into formal knowledge and finally codified into mechanisms of control such as job descriptions and incentive schemes [14–18]. Design thinking can be used during many stages in the maturation of innovation, and it can provide constructive means for managing tensions between grassroots and ivory towers.

9.4   Technology, Digitalization, and Work for Health

"There appears to be an imperative of possibility in healthcare. That which is possible to do has to be done" [19]. The ethos of inevitable and unquestioned technological progress is more generally known as *the technological imperative*.

Technological evolution seems to be propelled forward by almost uncontrolla-
ble forces.

Technology is *pulled* forward by needs of healthcare organizations as mediators
of the needs of patients and professionals, and technology is *pushed* by actors who
have stake in the medical technology market including established corporations,
nascent companies, researchers, developers, investors, opinion leaders, business
media, and so on. New technologies are being continually integrated into the practice of medicine. Technological adoption takes place at an intense rate, and some of
it is inappropriate. For example, there are unwise uses of technology that create
more distraction than ease for healthcare workers, and unwanted uses of technology
that disregard the autonomy of patients [19].

Healthcare can make use of an enormous range of different technologies.
However, even healthcare with all its scale and scope is affected by even larger
forces shaping the world. For example, over the past few decades, information technology has become ubiquitous with platforms and services expanding their reach to
most areas of life. The wave of economic transformation commonly referred to as
digitalization has brought about endless changes across all industries globally.

Digitalization has enabled enormous change and economic opportunity, and
therefore, much of design thinking discourse deals with digitalization. Also, especially in the early days of consumer Internet, much of new service concepts were
seen as amplifiers of individual freedom as well as communal and democratic
action, which as ideals served to attract interest from the design community.

However, design thinking does not imply nor necessitate *more digitalization*—it
only implies an attempt to identify the best possible solution. In the contemporary
technological world, it may not always be obvious what is *more* and what is *less*. An
application requiring a minimal input from a human user (seemingly less) may rely
on massively complex technological solution (actually more). Further, as technology becomes more and more ubiquitous and powerful, it becomes more like a com-
modity. Network and platform connectivity in its various meanings and modalities
has become a standard of the general infrastructure of knowledge work. Artificial
intelligence is on its way to becoming part of all data platforms. Amidst such
changes, the relationships between users, organizations, and technologies are continually re-negotiated. Those who are equipped with design sensibilities and methods have more to say in this kind of world. They are empowered by design thinking.

In addition to creativity, design thinking can facilitate constructive criticism,
which applies in the context of digitalization as well. Digitalization is a great
resource and opportunity, while at the same time digitalization can appear as a blank
canvas whereupon rather vague expectations are projected. The perspective of
design thinking—*inter alia* putting people in the center, questioning assumptions,
and looking for simple practical solutions—can provide healthy balance into considerations regarding the implementation of new technological solutions.

A word of warning is in place. Titular design thinking exercises and design-talk
have been integrated into the sales processes of technology providers. While engaging end-users, tailoring system specifications, and building commitment are well-
justified activities, vendor-driven design thinking might not always be the best

source of objectivity and creativity. In a cynical scenario design thinking is enacted as intellectually superficial *design theater* with the sole aim of packaging *more digitalization* based on technological assets in the vendor's repertoire.

Design thinking in healthcare shouldn't be moored onto technological assets, but, instead, it should be grounded on the *work for health* that people engage in. Isolated performance metrics (e.g., imaging resolution) of medical technologies are secondary to benefits they bring to the people they affect (e.g., a clinic as a workplace and the patients). Considering the chronic workforce shortage in healthcare, considerations regarding workflows and productivity are likely to become ever more prominent, which further emphasizes the value of human-centricity and the value of boots-on-the-ground practice and experience. Channeling that knowledge into decision making involves co-creation with all stakeholders and, in pragmatic terms, brings attention to patients as well as to healthcare workers as carriers of relevant information. It brings attention to the roles and workflows that structure the performance of work for health.

9.5   Design Thinking Practice for Future Healthcare

Instead of providing yet another conceptual simplification for appeasing administrative anxieties—some idealized framework for innovation management—design thinking offers methodology for purposeful experimentation and co-creation. It is a very practical approach for collaborating toward renewal.

Design thinking can have profound effects by bringing awareness to peoples' needs and expectations, and by questioning ideas that are taken for granted. It can be used to counter some of the rationalist hubris inherent in the centralized development of *socio-technical systems*. Healthcare needs design thinking to ensure that innovation has meaningful direction, and it serves ordinary people—patients and professionals alike.

This book provides many perspectives on design thinking in the context of healthcare. Yet, a single book can represent only a limited view of what key notions such as *healthcare* and *design* stand for across different cultures, societies, and economies. Many of this book's contributors are Finnish by birth. Many practical examples arise from the Finnish context, and they represent only a fraction of medicine and medical professions that have their specific sub-cultures and communities of practice. The reader should be aware of possible limitations to generalizability.

The most impactful way for utilizing this book (and many others like it) is to think how its recommendations and case studies might translate into the reader's own community and environment. So, instead of generalizing, the reader should focus on reflecting and translating, that is, finding ways for transferring ideas and approaches from one context to another. It is very conducive approach for learning; it can result in creative ideas, and it is a profound exercise in design thinking.

The formal knowledge presented on these pages should serve in building practical skills. The reader is encouraged into experimentation and reflection. It's about creating capabilities for having real-world impact based on one's own personal interests and insights. Reflecting upon one's own background, approach, and connections—"Who I am, What I know, Whom I know"—is key to identifying those very special change-making opportunities that would most benefit from a deep personal commitment for driving change (i.e., not only contributing to processes that are owned/driven/championed by other people) [1, 20].

Change in healthcare—and institutional change in general—is co-implicated with renewal of roles because institutions are upheld through the fulfillment of social roles [21]. Yet, no one is completely free to re-design their profession. Healthcare professionals are embedded in institutional structures. They have roles that involve assumptions and expectations that limit how opportunities for change are even identified, let alone valued. However, design thinking tends to challenge—nudge, shift, transcend—such limitations.

Design thinking can provide counterbalance to rationalist hubris, relentless supply push of technology, and precipitous medicalization. It relies on healthcare organizations not undervaluing the pragmatic and empathic know-how embodied in their staff and culture. Organizations that aspire true innovativeness and ethical leadership should be in the driver's seat of design. They cannot view design thinking as, for example, technology vendors' responsibility. Healthcare professionals should take charge as competent design thinkers. Indeed, integrating design thinking more deeply into healthcare education can unlock great potential.

The challenge of creating meaningful change within the existing medical system can appear overwhelming. Yet, answers are to be found through tackling practical issues, involving stakeholders early on, empathizing, and proceeding with grassroots experiments while recognizing existing structures and interests. Design thinking provides *tools and tradition* for these endeavors.

References

1. Sarasvathy SD (2022) Effectuation: elements of entrepreneurial expertise (new horizons in entrepreneurship series), 2nd edn. Edward Elgar Publishing, Cheltenham
2. Thornton PH et al (2012) Institutional logics perspective: a new approach to culture, structure, and process. Oxford University Press, New York
3. Scott JC (1998) Seeing Like a State: How Certain Schemes to Improve the Human Condition Have Failed. Yale University Press, New Haven
4. Barzelay M, Gallego R (2006) From "new institutionalism" to "institutional processualism": advancing knowledge about public management policy change. Governance 19(4):531–557
5. Capano G (2003) Administrative traditions and policy change: when policy paradigm matters. The case of Italian administrative reform during the 1990s. Public Adm 81(4):781–810
6. Drori GS, Meyer JW, Hwang H (eds) (2007) Globalization and organization: world society and organizational change. Oxford University Press, Cary
7. Hacker JS (2004) Dismantling the health care state? Political institutions, public policies and the comparative politics of health reform. Br J Polit Sci 34(4):693–724
8. Helderman J-K (2015) The crisis as catalyst for reframing health care policies in the European Union. Health Econom Policy Law 10:45–59
9. Lehto, J., Vrangbæk, K., & Winblad, U. (2015). The reactions to macro-economic crises in Nordic health system policies: Denmark, Finland and Sweden, 1980-2013

10. Windrum P, Koch P (eds) (2008) Innovation in public sector services: entrepreneurship, creativity and management. Edward Elgar Publishing, Northampton
11. Hacker JS (2005) Policy drift: the hidden politics of US welfare state retrenchment. In: Streeck W, Thelen KA (eds) Beyond continuity: institutional change in advanced political economies. Oxford University Press, Oxford, pp 40–82
12. Mattila Y (2011) Suuria käännekohtia vai tasaista kehitystä? Tutkimus Suomen terveydenhuollon suuntaviivoista. KELA, Helsinki
13. Teperi J et al (2009) The Finnish health care system: a value-based perspective. Sitra, Helsinki
14. Hasselbladh H, Kallinikos J (2000) The project of rationalization: a critique and reappraisal of neo-institutionalism in organization studies. Organ Stud 21(4):679–720
15. Hensmans M (2003) Social movement organizations: a metaphor for strategic actors in institutional fields. Organ Stud 24(3):355–381
16. Lindgren M, Packendorff J (2006) Entrepreneurship as boundary work: deviating from and belonging to community. In: Steyaert C, Hjorth D (eds) Entrepreneurship as social change. Edward Elgar, Cheltenham, pp 210–230
17. Sundin E, Tillmar M (2008) A Nurse and a Civil Servant changing institutions: entrepreneurial processes in different public sector organizations. Scand J Manag 24(2):113–124
18. Zilber T (2009) Institutional maintenance as narrative acts. In: Lawrence T, Suddaby R, Leca B (eds) Institutional work: actors and agency in Institutional Studies of Organizations. Cambridge University Press, Cambridge, pp 205–235
19. Hofmann B (2002) Is there a technological imperative in health care? Int J Technol Assess Health Care 18(3):675–689
20. Sarasvathy SD (2001) Causation and effectuation: toward a theoretical shift from economic inevitability to entrepreneurial contingency. Acad Manag Rev 26(2):243–263
21. Berger PL, Luckmann T (1967) The social construction of reality: a treatise in the sociology of knowledge. Anchor Books, Garden City